THE BIRCHALL DIET

A No Pills - No Frills Diet That is Easy to Follow

Stephen Birchall

authorHOUSE®

AuthorHouse™ UK Ltd.
500 Avebury Boulevard
Central Milton Keynes, MK9 2BE
www.authorhouse.co.uk
Phone: 08001974150

First published by AuthorHouse 1/22/2009

ISBN: 978-1-4389-4452-4 (sc)

Printed in the United States of America
Bloomington, Indiana

This book is printed on acid-free paper.

CONTENTS

INTRODUCTION

I had been seeing the scales gradually increasing and they reached a point where I decided that I <u>had</u> to lose weight, I didn't want to develop any health problems and I simply didn't like the way that my stomach was hiding my feet!

The problem I had was that there were far too many diets to choose from; I had no idea which diet would work best for me. They all had very impressive claims such as "easy to follow", "eat what you like", "lose 20 lbs in 20 days" etc. etc. so I could not choose a diet based on what they claim to do, because they all claimed to be the best diet available (and they can't ALL be right).

Some of the diets just sounded wrong for me because of the things I would have to endure. I enjoy my food and so there was no way that I was going to eat "Cabbage soups" or other weird combinations of foods that I simply don't like eating. Other diets relied heavily on exercise (I don't do "exercise! I have tried it and did not manage to keep it up for more than a couple of days). I did not want to have to keep charts, calculate points or examine food labels for content and calories etc. every time I wanted to eat something. In many ways I just wanted a "lazy person's" diet, a diet that allowed me to continue more or less as I currently do and just perhaps eat a little bit less than normal and still lose lots of weight. This seemed to be quite a tall order and nothing even came close (based on what I had heard from others or in the press etc.).

So even though there were plenty of diets around, there was nothing that I really connected with. I think that the main thing that seemed to be missing from virtually all of them was the fact that none of them seemed to fully explain the logic behind the diet. I felt that I had to understand WHY the diet worked rather than just IF it worked. I felt that it was important to understand the diet because I would have to change my lifestyle significantly for a long period of time and so I had to be sure that I was not going to waste my time. Also it would be having a major affect on my body and general health and well-being so I wanted to know exactly what was happening. I didn't want some unknown "expert" telling me that I should be eating X Calories a day or that a carrot is "X" points and a steak is "Y" points, or that I must eat foods low in "carbs", High in fibre etc.. How can they possibly know what MY body needs or how MY body processes different foods? After all, we may all be the same basic design but we are all (thankfully) unique, so what works for one person may well not work for another.

I thought about trying the "best selling" diets and even though some of them tried to explain why they work, I still couldn't relate them to me personally. They tended to base their concepts around the so-called "average" person; I want something that is based around me.

In addition to this I have yet to hear of a diet that works for everyone, if there was such as thing as the perfect diet, then why are there so many diets to choose from? How many times have you heard of diets that simply don't work? (You may have tried some of them already) How many stories have you heard about amazing weight loss and then heard that the weight just piled back on almost immediately? So I personally had no confidence in any of the diets I found, so I realised that I would have to develop one myself.

Another reason why I wanted to develop a new diet was due to the huge volume of complicated, unsubstantiated, conflicting advice from so-called "experts". Eat this, don't eat this, monitor your points, calories etc., the "low carb", "high carb", "low fat", "high fibre" diet and so on. If their advice conflicts in any way then they can't all be right and most DID conflict.

To me, one of the main problems with most diets is that they are overcomplicated and require you to believe the "expert" advice without explaining it to you fully enough to allow you to make up your own mind.

So I decided that the only option I had was to try to break the whole subject of dieting down to its basics and start with a totally clean sheet. I wanted to find a way to understand how the body works and how weight is gained and lost and use this as a basis for a new approach to dieting that uses common sense as its main principle. I wanted a diet that uses the amazing abilities that our bodies already have built in, so that it would be our body that controls our weight and not some "expert" telling us what is right for the "average" person.

When I started to develop my diet, I deliberately didn't set out to "tick all of the boxes" for what would be accepted as an "ideal diet". I didn't want to fall into the trap that other diets have fallen into, by looking at marketing claims and building a diet that sounds great but doesn't actually deliver results. I firmly believe that if the diet is based on the absolute basic functions of the body, how it works and what it actually needs to stay fit and healthy, then it would automatically "tick all of the boxes" anyway. I hope that you will agree that it achieves this when you have given it a try.

So to build a diet like this I decided to use my analytical skills (from my extensive computer systems design experience) and I always find that the best way to solve any problem is start with a "clean sheet" approach and not base it on anything I had seen or heard of before. I wanted to make sure that I started with no preconceived ideas about what a diet needs to do, no unproven "expert" advice, no "hearsay" (which is what most "expert advice" is in reality) and certainly no pills, strange foods or anything that I would not normally eat as a plain and simple human being. That way I could build a diet that does not base itself on anybody's theories; I could concentrate on common sense and simple facts and therefore ensure that everyone could understand WHY and HOW it works and therefore adapt it to their own unique requirements. I wanted a diet that everyone could follow and feel that THEY control what is happening.

The added advantage of the diet is that it can be used alongside many of the diets that you may be trying already because it is simply based on how we gain (and lose) weight. It has many tips and helpful explanations of how the body works and so you can use this in addition to any diet you are on, if you don't want to switch completely, or if you want to "pick and mix" the advice (although I believe that to obtain the best results you should try to follow this diet as closely as possible, of course). You can use this book to discover a little bit more about your body by looking at how it controls its own weight, from a fresh perspective. You can then take control of your own weight and use whatever diet you want to, knowing why and how it works.

I would suggest that after the diet has worked and you have hit your target weight, the book will help you to maintain your weight and even though you will be still following the principles of the diet you will not feel like you are on a diet. This will help you to ensure that you don't put the weight back on after all of the effort you have taken to lose it.

I have described the diet in depth in the following chapters but many of you might simply want to get started very quickly and then take time to read the details later. This is fine, I have summarised the main points here to get you started and there are some chapters that you need to read first if you really want a quick start.

Firstly I am not claiming to know the intricate workings of our bodies; we don't need to be biological experts to know the basic functions of our stomachs to enable us to lose some weight. We just need to understand how our bodies work at the very highest level, without going into any detail. I think many of the other diets on the market use this "mystery of the complexities of the body" and detailed analysis of food contents and simply confuse the issue. We are simply trying to reduce how much we eat; we do not need to make it much more complicated than that.

Let's look at the whole diet process from a completely different viewpoint and let's stay away from "expert" advice or special foods etc. for the moment.

Hopefully you will be able to agree with the following statements?

- The food and drink that we consume is basically the fuel our bodies need to operate.

- If we consume too much fuel our body will store the excess as fat to use later.

These are very basic statements but if you agree that they appear to be true (and I hope you can!) then we can use this as the basic information we need to enable us to control our weight.

Following the above statements, to reduce our weight we simply have to consume slightly less fuel than we need, so that our body consumes the extra fat that it has stored. I really cannot see why any diet needs to be more complicated than this.

One of the problems of achieving this is how to calculate how much to eat so that we do not starve, yet we consume our excess fat? Most diets try to guide you by stating how many calories, or how many points you should consume. The problem is that this depends on so many variables that it cannot be right for you specifically, especially since you might have had a very busy or a very lazy day. I believe that there is a simple method that we can use to manage the amount of food (fuel?) that we consume and it is a method that is VERY specific to you and you alone and it will vary automatically depending on how much energy you have used. We can use the signals that our body naturally uses to let us know exactly when to eat, and also how much to eat, we can use our "hunger sensation".

As soon as we feel the hunger sensation we IMMEDIATELY know that we are consuming the excess fat that we have in reserve. The hunger sensation is a signal that the body gives out to say "You better eat something soon, I am running on empty!" But this is EXACTLY what we are aiming for; we WANT to run on empty for a while to ensure that we consume our excess fat. So we WANT to feel hungry (at least for a while), if we are feeling the "hunger sensation" we are LOSING WEIGHT, it is as simple as that.

So basically if you are NOT feeling hungry (or at least "peckish") then you are NOT losing weight. This is where many diets fail, they give you ways to STOP the hunger sensation, they tell you to eat something with no points or with no calories etc. This DOES stop you from feeling hungry, but only because it stops your body from consuming the excess fat because it has been fooled into thinking that it has some "fuel" and so it stops using its reserves. This is the last thing we need if we are trying to burn off that excess fat that the body uses as reserve fuel.

This is the basis of this diet, plainly and simply, just allow yourself to feel hungry for a while before eating your next snack (or very small meal). The longer you feel hungry the more you will lose, but do not overdo it, you certainly don't have to starve yourself or make yourself feel very uncomfortable. Remember that you are just trying to lose a small percentage of your total weight, so you do not have to do anything drastic.

But when you do eat, remember that we want to "run on empty" and so just have a small meal or snack that will not fill you. What we are aiming for is to eat something that leaves you slightly peckish, avoid eating enough to make you feel full (or your body will store the extra as fat). When you do eat something, eat something "normal" avoid diet foods because your body NEEDS fuel, if you eat something "diet" you will rob your body of the energy it needs to enable it to operate correctly (and stay healthy). Eat something that you feel like but keep the portion size down so that you do not feel anywhere near full.

You will know IMMEDIATELY when you are losing weight, minute by minute, because you feel the hunger sensation, see this as a very positive signal when you are dieting and don't rush to suppress your hunger (as we are programmed to do quite naturally).

How hungry should you feel and for how long? Well it is vital (as I have already stated) to NEVER starve yourself, there is absolutely no need, we just need to reduce our fuel we do not need to overdo it, or we will damage our health.

As for how long should you allow yourself to feel hungry? This will be trial and error at first, but we have the advantage of weighing twice a day (more later on why this is important) and so we will be able to see if we are losing weight very quickly. But as a guide, the hunger sensation is deliberately uncomfortable because our body is warning us that we need to eat, so you will not want to be uncomfortable for long. But do try and stick with it, until you feel you have been uncomfortable for long enough. Don't worry though; it will become easier with time, especially when you see the scales falling.

You need to aim for a balance that means that the discomfort is matched by the weight loss you are seeing. It will be worth it believe me.

That is it! A diet does not need to be more complicated than that, although I have included lots of hints and tips on how to achieve your target weight quickly and easily in the following chapters. So if you want to get started straight away have a read through the "Basics of the diet", "The Golden rules" and a "Typical day" first. Then read through the rest of the book as and when you want to and hopefully you will be able to master your weight and feel totally in control within days.

The Author

At this point in the book it would be normal for the author to highlight the many qualifications they have in medicine, biology, health and fitness, science etc. but I do not possess these qualifications and I firmly believe that these qualifications are not necessary. We need a diet that we can all understand and "buy into", we are not all experts and so we need a diet that is easy to understand and one that makes plain and simply common sense. There are no qualifications available for "common sense"!!!!

So how can I expect you to follow a diet that has been written by someone without these qualifications?

The reason is that this diet is based on a basic understanding of how our bodies work. It is not based on detailed scientific principles that only an expert would know and understand. What is the point of me spouting detailed scientific statements if they are so detailed that only I would know if they were factual or not. My aim is to give you basic theories about how our bodies work and these are so basic that you should be able to agree or disagree with them yourself with no detailed scientific knowledge required. By doing this there should be no "mystery" involved and you should be able to understand exactly how to control your own weight using your own body and the signals it uses to achieve this.

I do, however, have experience that is relevant, but in computer system design. How is this relevant? In computer system design you have to solve very specific and often very complex problems. To achieve this you have to break these problems down to the basics to ensure that you have understood the problem, even if you are not necessarily an expert in the subject matter related to the problem. For example, I am currently working within the gas exploration business, I know nothing about gas exploration but I can determine the cause of specific problems by pure analysis of the facts and requirements. I then have to build a solution based on a "clean sheet" approach, it would be very dangerous to base any solution on assumptions and so I avoid this. I am a great believer in the adage that "if you ASSUME, you simply make an ASS out of U and ME!!!.

In many ways a diet is no different to a computer system problem; you still need to break the problem down to its basics first. We do this by understanding what is actually happening, such as "why do we put weight on anyway", "How do we put weight on", "How do we lose weight", "How does the body control weight naturally", "What foods make you overweight and why", "Why can some people eat large portions and not put weight on and yet someone else only has to have one square of chocolate and they put on weight?", etc. I have covered questions like these and more, in various chapters throughout the book.

I have been solving complex computer system problems by designing novel solutions for over 28 years now and I have written a "best selling" book on the subject. So I feel sufficiently qualified to attempt to solve the problem of finding a diet that works for each individual and relates to their needs specifically. I also have a high IQ (158), or so they tell me, which some people say is some kind of measure of intelligence. I am not saying this to impress anyone I just want to prove that I may have something to contribute to the solution.

One area that is vitally important whenever diets are developed is health, it would be very wrong of me to make medical claims and persuade people to do ANYTHING that could in any way affect their health in any negative way. This diet does not suggest that you change anything dramatically and it certainly does not suggest that you need to radically change your eating habits and so avoids many of the risks associated with some of the more complex or severe diets. The advice in this book is based on your normal body functions and if anything, it makes you more aware of warning signals etc. that are often ignored and should help to improve your overall health and well-being as well as your figure.

Hopefully you will be able to make up your own mind as to whether or not I have the appropriate knowledge to write this book. I sincerely hope that you will at least read the book and form your own opinions, but I am equally sure that your knowledge of how your body can control its own weight will at least help you, however you finally decide to diet.

WHY ARE YOU DIETING?

Before we start to discuss the diet in any detail, it is important to establish exactly why you want to lose weight, this has a major effect on how you should approach any diet.

Are you dieting for cosmetic reasons, for health reasons, or just because you think you should, for a special occasion, or to feel better about yourself etc.?

In fact these reasons actually break down into two main reasons, cosmetic and health.

If you are dieting just to feel better about yourself, this could be said to be cosmetic or health, it all depends on how overweight you are.

If you are only marginally overweight it could be that you just want to lose a bit of a "tummy", to me that would be cosmetic too.

If you don't feel good about yourself because of your body shape and it is affecting your confidence or making you feel low or depressed then this is probably better classed as being for health reasons, after all, your state of mind is vital to your health and if you are depressed then this is definitely a health reason.

One thing that always scares me is the fact that some people have the impression that they are overweight and they simply are not so PLEASE stop dieting when you hit your ideal Body Mass Index (BMI) range. If you try to lose weight and you don't need to you will seriously damage your health, check the various BMI charts that are readily available on the internet (you can also find these on my web site www.thebirchalldiet.com). I always maintain that you should only be aiming for the high part of "normal" or the low part of "overweight" on these charts. Please do not try to lose weight if your BMI already indicates that you are in the "normal" range, I feel that the BMI charts tend to indicate a slightly lower weight target than I would choose anyway.

So if you have decided which category you fall into then you have taken the first step to an improvement.

COSMETIC REASONS

If you are dieting for cosmetic reasons, i.e. to look better, to fit into certain clothes etc. then I MUST start with some warnings.

In no way do I want to stop you from dieting if that is what you really want to do, but dieting for cosmetic reasons does put you at risk health wise. The main reason for this is that we are very poor at judging our own image and it is so easy for us to THINK that we need to lose weight when we don't. Losing too much weight can be more dangerous than putting on too much weight. Illnesses such as Bulimia and Anorexia are life threatening, so PLEASE do try to follow the well-published guidelines as to the recommended minimum BMI etc. There are also many associations that specialise in illnesses like this, please to check out their web sites if you think that there is even a remote possibility of this happening to you. (See www.thebirchalldiet.com for some links to these important associations. I have deliberately not included these in the book because they can change over time and I will keep my web site up to date with any changes).

You need to have some extra weight in reserve to get you through any future illness you may experience. You must not have an "empty fuel tank" and have no fuel in the "reserve tank", this is very dangerous and even the smallest illness can become very serious if your body doesn't have the fuel it needs to fight it.

So please remember that the body NEEDS some extra weight to be stored for emergencies, imagine what would happen if you were at such a low weight that you had NO reserves of fat at all and then you contracted severe food poisoning or some other major illness, you would have no reserves of energy to help you get through this problem right at the very time when you need every once of energy and so it could even affect your survival.

I want this book to help people attain a HEALTHY weight, not just to lose weight, especially if they do not need to.

I am sorry to have to start in such a negative vein but I would not wish to be even remotely responsible for anyone suffering by trying to lose weight when they should not.

Lecture over (for now!).

HEALTH REASONS

I am sure that you have heard enough advice about being overweight and the medical risks that are associated with obesity, so I am not going to repeat these. This may be the very reason that you are prepared to try this (or any other) diet. But you don't have to be seriously overweight to suffer medical problems. One message that seems to be coming through loud and clear is that being even mildly overweight increases the risk of diabetes and other such illnesses. I am not in a position to question these findings (I am not a doctor) and so I fully support their advice to keep your weight within the recommended BMI range (or JUST above it).

Having said that being overweight is a risk, I do have to consider that there are people that have tried every diet available and failed and even some people that simply do not want to diet even if they are clinically obese. All I can do is to hope that these people can try my diet (if they want to lose weight) and gain some success, but the last thing that I want to do is to make people believe that they cannot make their own choices.

But hopefully you want to attain a healthy weight and are prepared to give this a try. If it works for you (as I hope it will), then perhaps it will help you feel better both mentally as well as physically.

It is quite natural for your body shape to change as you get older and so please don't damage your health trying to lose a "tummy" if your weight is already lower than it should be.

To sum up, please only diet if you are overweight (it sounds obvious but it really isn't unfortunately).

The Ideal diet?

By adopting a "clean sheet" approach to dieting this means that one of the first things we have to do is to establish what a successful diet should achieve. By producing this list we can then build a diet that "ticks all of the boxes".

I have deliberately avoided just reeling off a list of things that MY diet does, that would be dishonest and it would be blatantly obvious to you that I had done this. So I produced the list before I started developing the diet and constantly checked against it so that it would be the best diet I could design.

In my opinion the ideal diet -

- **Should be easy to follow** - There is no point in following a diet that is so complicated that it is easy to make mistakes. It is also not a great diet of you have to keep referring to charts and lists etc. every time you eat (especially if you are having a meal out, or with friends). Also if it is not easy to follow then perhaps this is an indication that it is not based on simple basic facts.

- **Must not be torture** - (although there is some truth in the "no pain - no gain" concept). For any diet to work you have to be able to stick with it. It has to have the right balance of results compared to the discomfort / effort involved.

After all, we could all simply stop eating and lose weight that way, but the pain would be unbearable and we would seriously damage our health.

- **Should not make me eat things I don't like** - there is no point in a diet that makes you eat foods that are unpleasant, you have to continue the diet for a long time and so this makes it hard to follow if you don't like what you have to eat. I believe that you should be able to diet using the foods you enjoy.

- **Should not be "anti-social"** - You should be able to follow a diet without appearing to be fanatical about it. For instance when eating out, or at family mealtimes etc. you should not have to give the host any special instructions or produce charts and guides at the table.

- **Should not involve charts / calculations / points etc.** - If the diet involves charts, calculations and or points then this (in my opinion) makes it cumbersome at the very least. Charts and calculations can be missed or updated incorrectly. If points or calories etc. are involved then it is often very difficult to establish the actual value of a meal etc. This can be especially inconvenient when you haven't personally prepared the food.

- **Should be suited to ME** - Diets that are built around the average person are never going to be ideal for everyone because we are not all average? The best diet for me would be one that allows for the way that I eat, work, exercise etc. and not just a "generic" person with a "generic" lifestyle. I want a diet that will change as I change. Even in a normal day my stress levels can change and this may well change the type and volume of food I need.

- **Should be flexible** - Life is unpredictable and we can never be sure of what will happen next, so I don't want a diet that is too rigid. I want to be able to modify the diet to suit my life. If I am lucky enough to visit a good restaurant then I don't want to have to choose a bland meal, I want to order what I like, after all this would be an exception. I also find that different days need different approaches, when I am busy at work I sometimes eat more due to stress etc. Other days I am so busy that I don't get chance to eat anything. I have more control of my food intake of a weekend and so I want a diet that can be different day by day.

- **Should clearly indicate when I am losing weight** - I don't want to have to wait until days later or even just hours later to find out if I am losing weight. My ideal diet would give me instant feedback minute by minute.

- **Should change my habits as well as my weight** - My ideal diet would help me to change my long term eating habits as well as my weight. I don't want to slip back into my bad habits after hitting my target weight.

- **MUST be healthy and should ideally make me MORE healthy** - A diet should consist of healthy foods that provide the energy my body needs to function correctly. I want to be healthier than I am now and stay that way.

- **Must not cost me any extra in food bills** - I don't want to have to pay more for my foods; I don't want to have to buy "special" or "diet" foods. I would prefer to be able to choose the food that I like and the foods that are readily available. In fact I would like to see a reduction in food bills if I am going to be eating less.

- **Should be a POSITIVE experience** - So that you can make it a part of your life. Even after you have reached your target weight you need to try to retain that weight and it is so much easier to follow a diet that you believe in.

- **Should not make me bulimic, anorexic or cause other health problems** - Some diets are quite severe and can lead to health problems, especially if they significantly change your habits. This diet is based on modifying the amount and frequency of your food and does not significantly change the type of food that you are used to eating. By making better use of your bodies signals (more of this later) you will be able to know when you are overdoing it. Having said this, the risks associated with ANY diet are important to monitor and understand.

- **Must not enforce exercise as a part of the diet (or prevent this if I enjoy it)** - There are many people that do not do enough exercise; however, I see this as a completely separate issue. Exercise is necessary to remain fit and healthy; I am not sure though that I would agree that it is categorically a vital part of a diet. Yes, one way to diet is to burn up more than you consume and so increasing exercise can be one way to burn up extra calories. But if you are forced to exercise as part of a diet and you really don't want to do that exercise then the diet will fail. I believe that we have to see the diet itself as a way to lose weight, if you can exercise as well, then this should be seen as a bonus. I personally exercise by playing golf every week, I enjoy it and I can do it regularly. I personally cannot manage to run on a machine or run through the streets, I even find it almost impossible to set aside a period each day to exercise in the home. So the diet MUST work even if exercise is not part of it. It must also not prevent me from exercising if I enjoy it.

- **Must not make me change my lifestyle in a negative way** - I MUST be able to fully enjoy my life as it is now, including meals out and parties etc. Without this I am not going to stick to the diet no matter how good it is. If I really feel like a steak with all of the trimmings then I must be able to do enjoy that. If the diet crumbles because of this then the diet is never going to work. The diet must help me understand the effects of my occasional "weaknesses" like this and how to recover from the occasional lapse. It must not ban any foods at any time.

- **Should be usable in all situations, at work, at home, dining out, on holiday etc**. - whereas some times the diet will be easier to follow than others, I must be able to follow it (at least in part) even when the situations change. If I go on holiday for instance, I would still like to enjoy my food but I would also like to at least be able to follow the principles of the diet.

- **Should make sense, I want to know why I am losing weight** - If I don't understand how the diet works I will not be able to follow it correctly. I have to be able to understand how and why the diet works so that I can manage my diet and vary it as and when I need to. The less "mystery" involved in the diet the more likely it is to succeed.

- **Should be something that I can continue even after I have stabilised my weight** - Once I have reached my target weight I don't want to feel that the diet ends there, I want to know how to retain my target weight, this can sometimes be as tricky as losing the weight in the first place.

- **Should be more "weight control" than diet** - A perfect diet should not be a "one-way street"; if a diet only helps you to lose weight then I am not sure that it is a good diet. I prefer a diet that is more a case of controlling weight rather then just losing it. If the principles of a diet are understood and are proved to have worked then it should be capable of helping someone retain a steady weight or even GAIN weight if they want to. I prefer a completely rounded solution; I want to feel as if I am in control of my weight. That way I can vary the amount of weight that I lose according to MY timetable.

- **Should give me quick results as well as long-term results** - I want to be able to lose weight quickly at first, then I would like to be able to continue to lose weight slowly until I reach my target weight. Losing weight too quickly can sometimes lead to it being put back on very quickly too, I would like to "educate" my stomach so that my weight stabilises.

- **Needs "will power" but this should not be excessive** - ANY diet will need to have an element of willpower, but I am only human I have moments of "weakness". I don't want a diet to succeed or fail, SOLELY on the strength of my willpower. I am prepared to try hard, but I cannot follow a diet that needs too much willpower from me.

- **Should not require any special equipment** - I have seen (or even tried) the various pieces of equipment that are seen on the "shopping channels", they seem so easy to use and the results that are promised are fantastic, but I have not yet succeeded in any way to get the results I was expecting. Exercise machines and similar equipment all need a large degree of willpower and commitment. I start with the best of intentions but fail soon after. Not only that but I have heard that muscle tissue is heavier than fat tissue and I just want to lose weight, I would like to look like a film star but it is just NOT going to happen. There is no problem with using the equipment if you already have it but as I have already said, this will aid your fitness and health more than your diet (so not a bad thing)

- **Should help me understand what has happened if I suddenly put on a few pounds** - This will happen, there will be times when your weight may increase slightly (perhaps you have been "naughty" and strayed from the guidelines). The most important thing is to understand why your weight has increased, how to get it down again and how long it will take. If we understand how the diet works we can then use this to understand what has happened and correct it.

- **Should enable me to vary the effects, sometimes just losing a bit and other times a lot** - I want complete control, sometimes I will want to push a bit harder and lose a bit more than usual and other times I might want to relax a little. I want a diet that I control and where I decide how much to lose and how.

- **Should not rob me of the pleasure of a enjoying a good meal** - There is nothing quite like a good meal, it is most enjoyable. I don't want to lose that altogether. I also might have to eat with friends etc. and I don't want to be the "odd one out". So I must be able to enjoy a meal if and when I like. The worst that should happen is that this should just temporarily slow down my weight loss; I should not feel as if I have broken the rules or lost my willpower.

- **Should allow me to eat a balanced diet** - I need to be able to eat a balanced diet, this includes some fats and sugars as well as some fibre, vegetables, salads etc. I do not want to switch to special or diet foods that are not wholesome or part of a balanced diet. I would rather eat "normal foods" and reduce the quantity than switch to totally new foods or low calorie versions of the foods I am used to eating. My health is vitally important to me and so I want to be able to eat foods that are good for me.

- **Must work for vegetarians and vegans as well as "meat eaters"** - If I was already a Vegetarian or Vegan I am not going to gain anything by cutting out the meat etc. that I don't eat anyway, so I would want a diet that works for me too. I would probably be already eating healthily; I would just want to lose weight.

- **Must be common sense so that I can understand it** - If I can understand how it works then I can follow it more closely and adapt it to suit my requirements. If I don't understand how it works I am more likely to make mistakes and be less successful.

- **Should not exclude chocolate, sugar or other treats** - I like my chocolate and biscuits etc. I would not like to have to ban them completely from my diet. As long as I know the effects I should be able to occasionally have a treat.

- **Should not make preparing meals more complicated** - I do not want meal preparation to be more complicated, especially if the rest of my family are not on the same diet as me. I want to be able to cook a meal that we can all have, I don't want to have to cook one meal for me and a different one for everyone else.

- **Must be proven to work** – A diet, however cleaver it seems must be proven to work, I don't want to invest a lot of time and effort for nothing.

- **Must not be like any of the other diets I have tried (and failed)** – There is no point in me trying a diet that is similar to ones that I have already tried and failed. It must be something different.

- **Must not enforce attendance at regular meetings** – I don't want to have to go to meetings or "weigh ins" if I don't feel like it. I want to diet in my own time and when it is convenient for me.

- **Should "educate my stomach" so that the weight loss stays off** – If I want to lose weight now then I surely don't want to put it back on. I want to change my eating habits in the long term. I don't want to over-eat, I would like to eat normally and feel as if I have eaten enough with normal sized portions.

- **Should ideally reduce the areas where my fat has built up and not affect some other areas quite so much** – I want to lose weight where it shows, I don't want to lose too much weight from areas that I don't believe are fat anyway. Ideally I would like to lose my stomach fat first.

Your body, what it is capable of?

Your body is truly amazing, but we take it for granted, often because we simply do not stop and think about what is actually happening.

The most amazing thing of all is the way that our body can produce a completely new life (or at least contribute to the process if we are mere males!). Stop and think about this for a moment, it can actually reproduce; it can grow all of the organs, hair, teeth, eyes etc. etc. a complete human being, how amazing is that?

Some lesser, but still amazing abilities include the ability to repair itself, it can heal cuts, mend broken bones, kill off bacteria and fight many diseases etc.

On a more relevant vein, it can carry out a LOT of physical and mental activity (just think how active you are in a busy day) and yet be powered by nothing more than a few sandwiches and a drink. It is the ultimate is fuel efficiency. This is very relevant to this whole diet; we are going to be looking at how the body manages to control the amount we eat, when we eat it and how we store any excess.

Let's imagine that we have a group of the best scientists available and we ask them to build a robot. They can, and already have, done this in varying degrees, but compared to a human being their skills and abilities are very limited, yet they consume a huge amount of power. A sandwich and a cup of tea are not going to power it for long (probably just long enough to switch itself off immediately after being switched on!).

So we will concentrate on just one element of this, the element that is most relevant to a diet, the stomach and how it works. This should help us understand about what, when and how to eat, so that we can ensure that we make full use of the inbuilt abilities of our body and use its ability to control our weight.

We must think of our stomach and complete digestive system as being our fuel tank and any extra fuel is stored in reserve tanks spread around our body - our fat! This means that we need to focus on one thing only and that is reducing the amount of fuel that we carry in reserve. We need to determine how to empty our reserve fuel tanks and stop them from being over-filled again. Our body will quite naturally try to keep our main fuel tank full and store any excess in our reserve tanks for use in emergencies (where food is scarce). But in modern times it would be extremely rare for us to find ourselves in a position where we could not access food for days on end (unlike our ancestors who were not so lucky). So we do not need to maintain large reserves of fat and there is no reason to have full reserve fuel tanks. The fact that food is now so readily available is one of the reasons why in recent times people seem to be getting more and more overweight. Our ancestors often had times when food was scarce and other times when food was plentiful (after we managed to kill an animal etc.) so they HAD to have a means of storing a large quantity of excess food (fuel). In modern times we can normally find wholesome food wherever we go and so we don't have to store so much, but it is so convenient that our bodies seem to just keep taking it in and storing it for "lean" times, which never come.

Throughout this book I will be referring to this process of storing food as fat as reserve fuel and as such, it does form the basis of the diet.

As far as the body is concerned it is easily capable of converting food to fuel and storing any excess as reserves. But to control this and make sure that WE decide how much extra fuel we want to carry we have to feed it the right fuel and in the correct proportions. Give it too much and it will fill up the reserve tanks and keep on filling them. This will continue for as long as we keep overeating, there is virtually no limit to the extra fuel we can store. Once we get past a certain point it will start to affect our health but many years ago before convenience foods, this would never happen. Once someone became too large, their ability to hunt and collect food was naturally impaired and so they became less efficient at finding food and so they burnt off their excess fuel. These days you don't have to exert any energy to obtain food and so we have lost the self regulation that we have had for many thousands of years.

So I believe that our body has the ability to self-regulate its own weight as long as we bear in mind the modern times we live in and avoid the problems associated with ease of access to food.

In the next section we will look at the signals and messages that our body gives out that can enable us to help it to self-regulate our weight.

Signals / Warnings

Our body has many signals and warnings that we sometimes ignore. If we get a headache we take a tablet, which then eases the headache. But the problem is that the headache was a warning and by switching that warning off with a tablet, we are ignoring that cause of the pain. Luckily enough it is often just a minor warning and so switching it off in this way does not normally cause us any lasting harm. But switching off or ignoring any signals and warnings that our body sends out is not something that we should do lightly.

In the previous section we discussed how amazing our bodies are and these signals and warnings are yet another example of its amazing capabilities. I tend to respect these signals and try to understand them because I believe that they are vital if we are to allow our bodies to carry on doing what they do well.

The signals and warnings that we are focussing on here though are those that relate directly to our diet. We have already mentioned the fact that we have a main fuel tank (our stomach) and reserve fuel tanks (our fat) and the signals that we need to watch out for relate to these. So in fact we are looking out for Fuel tank signals.

One that we are probably used to is the feeling we get when we are "full" after a meal. This feeling is quite pleasant and yet a little uncomfortable. This is our body's signal to tell us that the main fuel tank is full, stop eating. It has given us pleasant signals as a reward for eating a hearty meal, but it then has to give us some discomfort to indicate that we should stop.

The other main signal is the one that is absolutely central to this diet and that is the signal that we think of as being hungry. If we can master this signal and use it to our advantage we can gain full control of our weight.

We all experience this hunger sensation and we all believe this to be a clear indication that we are "hungry" and so we eat something. The hunger sensation is quite uncomfortable and we often eat something straight away so that we never feel hungry for long.

In effect it is ALMOST correct to think of this as a trigger to eat something, but it is (in my view) one of the main reasons why most diets fail. I believe that this signal is not simply a signal for us to eat something. I believe that it is a sensation that we experience when we are consuming some of our reserve fuel and so in a way it IS a signal that we should eat something. You would expect to feel very differently when your body switches to digesting your stomach fat wouldn't you. That is EXACTLY what I believe the signal to be. It is NOT a signal to eat something; it is a sensation that tells us that we are consuming our reserves. In the bad old days this definitely WOULD be a signal to eat something and quite quickly, because we would be running low on reserve fuels and we would have to find food (which could take a long time back then). But since we do not need so much reserve fuel these days, because food is so readily available, we should not be responding so quickly to this signal.

Not only that, but if it really IS a signal that our body is consuming our reserve fuels then this is EXACTLY what we want to do if we want to lose some weight. So instead of immediately responding to this signal and eating something, we should be allowing it to continue for a short while so that we can burn some reserve fuel and therefore get rid of some fat.

It is easy to see why we get this signal confused and think of it as "hunger" because it does mean that we should consider eating something. Our body has developed over thousands of years based around the fact that food is hard to come by and so when the reserves start to be consumed it is not surprising that our body sends out signals to try to get us to eat. But once we have realised EXACTLY what this signal means we can use this to control our weight more easily. We can use it as an instant indication of exactly when we are losing weight; we don't have to wait for the scales to tell us. As soon as we feel this sensation that we call "hunger" we know that we are losing weight, so see it as a very positive signal and not a negative one. This may take a few days to get used to, our natural reaction is to find a way to stop these sensations, but if we can put up with this slight discomfort for at least a short while we will lose weight.

What you must NOT do, is to starve yourself, you do not need to go without food to the extent that you are experiencing full hunger pains. Just allow yourself to feel this hunger sensation for a short while before you eat something.

So this is the main part of this diet, use this signal to know exactly when you are losing weight and don't artificially suppress it with diet foods, zero point foods, water etc..

Thirst / Hydration

In addition to the fuel we need, we have to ensure that we have enough liquids. Our body contains a lot of water and it is vital to retain this balance.

Our body, once again, can control this for us as long as we "listen" to the signals we get and understand them.

If we concentrate on the simplest of liquids for now - water, we can discuss other drinks later, but they are all based on water in one way or another.

There are lots of experts suggesting that we should all drink more water and they are PROBABLY right, but a recommendation to drink X litres of water a day cannot surely be correct? Everyone is different and even if we weren't what we do, what we eat or what we drink each day varies dramatically and so there cannot be a single recommendation for how much you should drink.

Once again, if we look way back in history, water was nowhere near as readily available as it is today (not to mention the quality of what was available). So I believe that we have to make sure that we are not using yesterday's needs in today's society. I DO listen to ONE expert and that is my body!

Providing that we are not unwell, we have an inbuilt mechanism for controlling how much water our body has, this is simply called "thirst". If our body is low on liquids we feel thirsty, this is our body sending out signals to us to persuade us to drink something. The main difference between liquids and food is that if we drink more than we need our body does not store it in specific areas like it does with our reserve fuel tanks. It absorbs it into the body generally and so our fluid retention varies. This has a direct affect on our weight and so over drinking can be as responsible for us being overweight as over eating is. There is one big difference though, our body can get rid of excess fluids much more easily and quicker than it can get rid of excess food (how many times a day do you visit the toilet and how many times is that to urinate?).

There are many verified reasons why it can be very dangerous for you to become dehydrated, so you MUST try to retain the correct level of liquids. But this should be easy enough just by using our body's abilities to self regulate itself.

Thirst, is a sensation that our body uses when it senses that we need more fluids. So as long as you are not ignoring this sensation (and you must NEVER ignore it) you should find that you are not going to dehydrate (and certainly not enough to cause you any medical problems). So when you feel thirsty (even slightly thirsty) have something to drink. Water is fine, but tea and the occasional coffee are fine too. Fruit juices are good in many ways but if they contain any artificial flavourings or sugar substitutes then you have to be careful, sometimes these leave an aftertaste and this CAN be mistaken for thirst (your body is actually signalling that you need to wash away that residue somehow, it is not the same as thirst). For these reasons I don't personally drink diet drinks and especially if they have artificial sugars / sweeteners. I simply do not like the aftertaste. I prefer fresh fruit juices etc. or just water. After all, the signal your body is giving you is thirst, i.e. it needs liquids (not chemicals).

Watch how much you drink, you do not have to have a full can or bottle of drink, often a few sips can be enough to satisfy your thirst. We often get into the habit of finishing the can or bottle and who designed the volume of the can / bottle? The manufacturer decided how much to put in the can / bottle and this is more likely to be based on their economics rather than a recommended amount to drink

Water and any fluids are heavy, one litre of water weighs one kilo (around 2.2 lbs) and if you are on a diet you have to consider this and so drinking too much is pointless. So if you are thirsty - drink! If you are not thirsty - don't drink!

Don't just drink X litres a day because someone has indicated that this is good for you. Some people lose more fluids than others and so your needs will vary, rely instead on your body signals to control your liquid intake.

Many people put on weight after going out for a meal at a restaurant and quite obviously blame the food, but consider how much liquid you had and you may be surprised to find that it could be that the drink added far more weight than the food did.

Let's say that you have a drink or two at the bar first and then you have some wine with the meal, some water as well, followed by coffee and a liqueur of some kind? (Not to mention the liquid in the dessert). That could be as much as two litres and probably more, but two litres weighs two kilos (approx four and a half pounds). Compare that to the weight of the food and are you sure that it is the meal that is responsible for the added weight???

Fuel for your engine

We have to remove all of the theories, "expert" opinions and preconceived ideas about food; we need to look at the absolute basics so that we can understand how our own body works and what we have to do to control OUR diet to match OUR requirements.

Basically your body needs food to give it the fuel it needs to operate. The amount of fuel your body needs varies dependant on what you are doing. If you are very active it needs more fuel than if you just sit there doing nothing, but whatever happens it needs "fuel".

If you consume too much fuel your body will store this as fat reserves to use later when food may not be available (think of this as a reserve fuel tank). If you consume too little fuel you will force your body to consume the fat reserves it has built up.

So as you can see this is how we can control our weight. We need to make sure that we are not ADDING any fuel reserves (this is the opposite of what we are trying to achieve). To avoid adding fat reserves we need to make sure that we do not consume too much fuel.

Be careful though, fuel is NOT the same as food because different foods have different amounts of fuel in them, ranging from water (with virtually zero fuel, but with other benefits) to a thick juicy steak with strips of fat on it (maximum fuel value). Because different foods contain different amounts of fuel, you will need different quantities of food depending on what you are eating. For example, you may find that a tiny mouthful of steak will give you a similar amount of fuel as a VERY large salad.

This is where many diets focus on calories and points etc. and some diets develop lists of foods that you must avoid. The reason that they do this is so that you limit the amount of fuel that you eat and this is to attempt to get you to a point where you are consuming less fuel than you need, so that your body burns off the excess fat that you have stored. The problem with this approach is that we are all different and we are all doing different things each day and so there really is NO ideal level of fuel, it all depends on one thing and that is YOU and what you have been doing. In addition to this, how can we possibly be expected to determine how many calories are in everything we eat and how many calories we are burning? Using charts and reading labels will help, but many foods are not labelled and it is impossible to know how much we are burning accurately. So I feel that there should be a better way of getting this "fuel balance" that we need. I think we should use something designed to do this, our own body and its signals.

Before we start looking at how we can use our own body signals to ensure that we do not have too much fuel we need to look at why many diets ban certain foods. Sugars and fats and high calorie foods are banned by many diets and avoided by most of the others. I believe that this is WRONG (from a diet viewpoint), these foods are basically no different to other foods apart from one simple fact, they contain a HIGH proportion of fuel (you can call this calories but I prefer to keep it much simpler than that).

As far as our body is concerned, as we have already said, if we consume too much fuel it will be stored for use later (as fat). So whatever you are eating, the amount of fuel matters MUCH more than the type or quantity of the food you are eating.

Yes, sugars and fats etc. are something that we have to be very careful with, but ONLY because of the high proportion of fuel that they contain (and any health reasons). By banning foods like this from any diet we are actually (in my opinion) removing a very important option we have to reduce the VOLUME of food we eat (and therefore reduce our stomach capacity).

Consider this, if we were trying to eat slightly less fuel than we need (as I hope you agree is the approach we need to take?) so that we can lose weight, which would be best? To eat a food that is low in fuel or high in fuel? I would say we should be eating something that is HIGH in fuel but low in volume. That way we can get exactly the same amount of fuel but with a much reduced quantity. If we were to go with the food that is LOW in fuel, we would need to eat a LOT more of it to give our body the same amount of fuel (i.e. just less than we need).

If we eat large volumes of food that is low in fuel, our stomach will expand to be able to handle this volume and this is the opposite of what we want.

So eating diet foods that are low in fuel will result in consuming larger volumes.

Remember that the important thing is to consume less fuel than we need, but still enough fuel to allow our body to operate correctly. You have a choice as to what food you eat to give you that fuel, so choose something that your body is telling you that you need rather than something that is deliberately low in fuel. Your body will need different foods at different times so "listen" to the signals and eat the food that you are craving, that way you are likely to eat less.

One of the main problems on any diet is knowing how much to eat of whatever food you have decided to consume. We do not want to have to have charts etc, or try and determine the fuel value of the food we are eating; this makes the whole process too messy and makes the diet more difficult to follow. To keep this simple we just need to know the major food types and if they are high in fuel or not, we can then use our judgement as to how much we should eat. This does not have to be super-accurate because we will be following our other main guideline of eating little and often anyway. In addition to this if we were to have a little bit more fuel than we should have it will just mean that it will be a little bit longer before we feel hungry again and so this becomes self correcting. Our portion size should never be large enough to result in us eating enough to enable our body to store any extra as fat reserves anyway. I simply never eat enough to feel full, if I can eat something and still feel a little peckish afterwards then that is perfect.

So which foods are high in fuel, this should be easy enough to establish, these are the foods that most diets suggest that you leave alone. Sugars, foods that contain butter / fat / cream etc. they are well known as being high in fuel (calories?). Meats are the one fuel type that has an extra element to consider, not only are they very high in fuel, but they are very solid and so release this fuel over a long time (they stay in your digestive system for a long time and this also adds weight while they are in there) but they are a high grade fuel.

Sugar is a strange food in many ways, even the "experts" often say that sugar by itself does not cause you to increase your weight, it contains no fat and after all, it is vegetable based (sugar cane?). So why is sugar seen as being responsible for weight gain? Could it be that it is VERY high in fuel and so when it is mixed with other foods it means that the result is that your body has consumed more fuel than it needs and so it stores the accompanying food as fat reserves instead of just consuming it? In addition to this, because it is so high in fuel, your body can burn this fuel off instead of burning off the reserves of fat it has stored, thereby slowing down your weight loss.

So treat sugar as a high grade fuel and if you have any (in the form of chocolate or anything else) just reduce the quantity you eat. A couple of pieces of chocolate are fine for a snack and will keep you going until the next snack.

In summary, think of the amount of FUEL that you are eating in a snack and try to ensure that you are eating slightly less than you need so that your body can burn up the reserve fat. If you can eat a snack or meal and still feel slightly hungry after it then this is perfect, you have given your body some fuel that it needs and yet you are still burning off excess fat.

But the most important thing that you need to do is to avoid eating enough fuel to enable your body to store any as reserve fuel. One of the main ways of achieving this is to ensure that you never feel full, especially at meal times. Just have small snacks throughout the day and slightly larger snacks at mealtimes.

How the laws of science apply to your weight

I am not going to get too technical / scientific at this point but I do think that we need to think about some really basic laws of science that are generally accepted as fact. it is easy to develop assumptions about what happens when we eat and it is best to dispel these assumptions because they can mislead us and this can affect how successful our diet is.

The most basic of these laws of science is the fact that weight (mass) does not just magically disappear or appear. If you eat something that weights one kilo it will increase your weight by one kilo, no more and no less, no matter what it was you ate. For example, if you eat a half kilo of steak it will add exactly the same weight as if you drink half a litre of water (one litre of water weighs one kilo).

All of the time that the steak / water stays in your body, it will add to your weight. The steak will not magically be increased or decreased in weight. This is a law of science however unlikely it seems.

Using this same basic principal, adding two spoons of sugar in your tea / coffee can only add (as a maximum) the weight of two spoons of sugar, it does not magically increase your weight by more than its own weight.

The scientific law states that "the mass of a closed system will remain constant, regardless of the processes acting inside the system". This means that the weight of the food you have eaten cannot be increased or decreased just by what happens in your stomach.

Another way of wording this is that "matter cannot be created/ destroyed, although it may be rearranged. This implies that for any chemical process in a closed system (i.e. our digestive system), the mass of the reactants must equal the mass of the products". This means that although the food we have eaten may well be broken down, but all that is happening is that anything that is lost from the food is simply converted to other substances that are also still in the body and so there is no weight loss. It is often converted to liquids and lost via urine and that is how the weight is "burnt off".

What does this mean and how is it relevant?

It means that your weight is only <u>ever</u> increased by the weight of the food you eat; there is no way that anything adds to that weight just because the food you ate contained sugar or fat etc.

So one kilo of ANY food will add the same weight as one kilo of water. The difference is purely down to how much of that food is retained by the body and how much is passed out (via sweat or the toilet!). We therefore can use this law to determine exactly how and why we gain or lose weight. There is no magic or mysterious process. If we are gaining weight, then it is simply because we are putting more food into our body than we are getting rid of. If we can agree with this we can therefore look at the type of foods that we eat and try to eat those foods that do not leave as much behind as others and so not build up our body weight any more than we have to.

This leads to one of the golden rules, and that is the guideline that we follow on this diet that helps us decide what foods to eat. This is the "squashable / dilutable" guide and it is one of the main principles of the diet. By following this guideline we are consuming foods that the body can process very quickly and therefore get rid of it very quickly. If a food can be squashed easily AND it can be diluted, then your digestive system will be able to process is more easily and the majority of it can be expelled from the body as urine, very shortly after eating it. This means that the weight of the food we ate is lost very quickly and the body does not have chance to extract all of the fuel from it.

If the food cannot be squashed easily AND if it cannot be diluted easily then it will take a long time to digest (and so the weight of this food will show up on the scales while the food stays in your body). Very little of this is expelled as urine and so the impact of this is felt for a long while and the body can extract all of the fuel from that food over a long period.

So basically science gives us the fact that the mass (weight) of any food that you eat cannot just increase or decrease, it will either be expelled from your body or kept "on board", so if we eat foods that can be easily expelled it is far better than solid foods that are carried for a long time. Fatty and sugary foods are only bad for a diet because they can cause more fuel to be stored in your reserve tanks. (Fatty foods are easier to convert to fat reserves and sugary foods are high in fuel value and so the body uses fewer reserves and can store more fuel from the accompanying food.) It is NOT because sugar or fat multiplies the weight of the food in any way.

If you want to lose weight, exercising does not actually burn up the food you have eaten, as such, it does not just disappear; science dictates that this weight can only be lost via sweat (only a small amount of course) or down the toilet. It is important to realise that weight is just not burnt up and weight is not increased due to the type of food you have eaten (i.e. adding sugar does not increase your weight by anything more than the weight of the sugar).

Understanding this basic law of science can help you understand the effects of food on your weight and help you to control it better.

FOOD LIKES / DISLIKES? WHAT IS ACTUALLY HAPPENING?

This is one of the questions that probably caused me to develop my diet in the first place; it was something that I never really thought to analyse in any depth. After all, we all know exactly what we mean when we say that we like or dislike the taste of something, don't we? Just think about this for a while and try to put it into different words, can you describe what you mean when you say you "like" something? The nearest thing is saying that it makes you feel good perhaps?

I am not so sure that we DO understand what we mean when we say that we like or dislike certain foods. To prove that we don't REALLY understand this, I would ask if you could explain what you mean when you say that you like a certain food, chocolate for example.

I started off by describing it as "when I start eating chocolate, it tastes nice, VERY nice" but that in itself is not an explanation. What do we mean by "it tastes nice" and why do some things taste nice and other things taste horrible?

We have to break this down into something far more basic than simple likes and dislikes. If we consider a subject that we covered earlier in the book and that is how very special our bodies are and how our body is very "clever", this could help us to understand this feeling we have called pleasure, like, dislike etc.

I believe that our body is clever enough to issue "rewards" when we do things that are good for us. Leaving aside the complex nature of our emotions and love etc. and looking at something far more relevant, our digestive system, we will see that these rewards are very relevant to our diet.

The next time you feel hungry, stop for a moment and think about the feelings you are experiencing. Your hunger is normally for specific types of food, you normally "feel like" something sweet, or something savoury, something dry or something liquid. In fact our hunger is far more specific than this, we quite often "feel like" very specific foods at different times. I don't think that we EVER just feel hungry, we always feel a hungry for something specific. This is our body's way of obtaining the appropriate food, chemical, vitamins etc. that it needs to balance itself.

For example, sometimes after drinking a beer we feel like a packet of crisps, a packet of peanuts, a pizza, kebab etc. There is a reason for this very specific hunger, our body has detected that we now have an excess of liquid and it is trying to balance the contents of our stomach. It does this by sending out messages to the brain to encourage you to eat that specific type of food. It then issues "reward" signals when you actually eat the correct food. This is why you use the expression "I feel like ....".

So I firmly believe that we can let our body tell us what we should eat, if we feel like eating a certain food, that is for a reason and so we should actually try to eat specifically that type of food. When we say that we like or dislike a food this is because our body is telling us what it wants us to eat or not to eat. So every time we ignore this specific hunger signal and eat something else, we are "cheating" our body and may find that this results in us eating more just to satisfy the body's needs.

These likes and dislikes can appear to be random, but I believe that there is a very logical reason behind all of our likes and dislikes when it comes to food. For instance, I have one unusual "dislike" and that is that I REALLY do not like salads and vegetables, therefore I simply do not eat them by choice. I have no idea why this is but I genuinely and absolutely dislike the taste of virtually all vegetables and most salad foods. This is a genuine dislike it is not me purely being fussy.

I am simply getting signals from my body that it does not want these foods. Vegetables and salads provide a lot of essential vitamins and minerals etc. (or so I am told) and so I guess that I must be getting these from something else.

I have read somewhere that some people have an acute sense of taste and it is possible that these people are able to taste minute (relatively harmless) poisons that are present in many vegetables. Whether this is true or not I am not sure, all I know is that I simply do not like the taste and so I don't eat them, I would never eat anything I didn't like the taste of (I suppose that medicines may be an exception).

I believe that my body is able to determine exactly what I should and shouldn't eat, within reason, so I am guided by it.

So in other areas of this book when I say that you should eat what you like or crave, I mean this absolutely. Your body is sending out signals to get you to eat something very specific, if you ignore this and eat something else (a diet food of some kind perhaps), your body will STILL need what it was asking for and you will end up eating more than you needed to.

Eating what you feel like is basically eating what your body needs.

So if you can now understand what is happening when you say that you like or dislike something, then you are well on the way to controlling your weight by listening to your body.

One thing that you have to be careful of is that you also have a memory and this can sometimes trick you, especially if you are not listening to the signals from your body closely enough. Let's take our good old friend - chocolate, as an example. One of the reasons that many of us like chocolate so much is that it is a really high grade fuel for our body, it contains fats, sugars and milk etc. and this is probably one of the highest grade fuels that we can find. This means that on the occasions where we were hungry in the past and ate some chocolate, our body would have given us some serious reward signals for this. This would have made us feel VERY good.

If we get these rewards regularly, we get used to them and if we are feeling low and want to feel good our memory bank recalls the pleasure we had when we ate chocolate. So it is entirely possible that we might THINK that we feel like some chocolate, when we actually are feeling like the sensation that we had when we ate chocolate in the past.

This is why we have to listen more closely to the signals that come from our stomach, than those that come from our memory. So the next time you think that you feel like chocolate, make sure that it is because your HUNGER signal indicates that you need something sweet like this.

If you can determine the difference between the two (your memory and your hunger) then you are now in control and can decide to eat whatever is right for you at that specific time.

So the next time your hunger tells you that you feel like something very specific please do have exactly that, don't just grab something with less fuel (calories) or a diet option, you should try to match your hunger precisely. Just be careful about the quantity you eat rather than what you eat, I really do believe that your body knows best.

STOMACH SIZE AND CAPACITY

In this context by stomach size I mean the size of the actual stomach, not your waist size or belly (we can deal with that later).

If our stomach has a large capacity it can process more food, it can hold more food (and therefore more weight) and it takes more food to satisfy our hunger, or feel full. In addition to this the stomach acid is spread further and is less strong and so it takes longer to process food than normal.

So in short, a large stomach capacity is wrong in so many ways, anything we can do to reduce this is going to pay dividends in the short and, more importantly, the long term.

But how do we manage to reduce our stomach size? The main way to achieve this is to "educate" your stomach. This can be done by reducing the volume of food that you are eating and sustain that reduction for a period of time. Most diets SAY that they are going to help you eat less but in fact they can often do the opposite, especially if they try to get you to eat foods that are lower in calories, smaller in points, or just plain "diet". This is because the foods may well have less fuel in them but the volume itself can be extremely large. A couple of pounds of carrots have (according to most diets) zero points and so you can virtually eat as many as you like, but carrots are heavy and the volume can be large and so they are not that good for a diet, regardless of the points.

The reason why I say this is because food that is low in calories / points or is diet contains greatly reduced fuel for your body. But your body will still need to have SOME fuel to allow it to operate, if that fuel is provided by low calorie / low points or diet foods then you have to eat a lot of it to get the minimum fuel you need. The increase in volume that is required to achieve the basic fuel needs will have an effect on the size of your stomach. It has to grow to handle the extra volume.

One way to reduce the size of your stomach is to avoid low calorie / points, diet foods as much as possible. By eating "normal" foods in smaller than normal quantities, you are able to match the same fuel levels as with diet foods, but the total volume is dramatically smaller. This allows your stomach to shrink down over time as it gets used to dealing with smaller volumes. This in turn enables you to feel full quicker and thereby reduce the volume of food that you need to eat. Your smaller stomach will hold less food (and therefore less weight on the scales), it will take up less space (and so reduce the inches), it should also be more efficient at processing the food and this would enable food to pass through quicker. All in all it is a "win win" situation.

I find that after following the diet for a few weeks I have educated my stomach to expect less volume and my hunger sensations are easier to manage. This will mean that I can follow the principles of this diet for as long as I want to and I am much less likely to go back to the old eating (overeating) habits.

WHAT IS AN IDEAL WEIGHT?

Firstly, there is no such thing as an ideal weight, we are all different and some people are larger than others.

Some people stay slim all of their lives, others stay large. I prefer to look at in a different way; simply that there are weights that should be avoided for health reasons.

You should aim to be at a weight that is right for YOU.

You know your normal body size, this has been your size for many years, if you have been grossly overweight all of your life an ideal weight for you would be to aim to lose enough weight to make you more healthy and make you feel happier with your shape; there is no point aiming to reach some theoretical body weight on a chart if all that is going to happen is that you feel as if you have failed just because you didn't lose enough weight.

If you can lose SOME weight, ANY weight, this should be seen as a step in the right direction. Be proud that you have lost weight and see it as positive. See it as proof that the diet works, don't just see it as enabling you to eat more now that you have lost some weight. If you have set a target weight, however aggressive, you will only feel really good when you have reached that target, so do not have an ideal weight in mind if this is not one that you absolutely believe that you will be able to achieve.

To me, an ideal weight will always be one that is slightly heavier than your target. There are two reasons for this, firstly your weight will always fluctuate and if you set a target and aim for and achieve that exact weight, you will always be just over it just under it, as your weight naturally varies. This will mean that you will not know whether to try to lose that couple of pounds or not. Secondly you can never tell when you might need those extra few pounds; after all they are your reserve fuel tank. You may be struck down with a stomach bug or other illness where you need every ounce of strength to stay well. If you have zero reserve fat you may find that you are unable to fight off this illness and may suffer for that.

So an ideal weight is one that is slightly more than your target. This target will vary with age, as you get older your body shape will naturally change and this is something that you should not try to fight to such an extent that you harm your health. The truth is that as you get older you are more susceptible to major illnesses and therefore your body will naturally try to store extra fuel in reserve for any such crisis. People often talk about "middle age spread", this is often just the body's way of preparing itself for problems. It is just your body's way of protecting you and so you should not try to fight it too hard. This doesn't mean that just because you are getting older that you cannot or should not diet; it just means that you should bear this in mind and perhaps not try to achieve your ideal weight (or shape) at all costs. A bit of a "belly" as you get older is not the same as having a bit of a "belly" when you are in your prime.

You will see lots of BMI charts and they all have a "band" that is where you will be classed as "normal" (I HATE that word in this context), "Overweight", "Obese" etc. I believe that if you are on the heavy side of normal or the light side or overweight then you are pretty much at your ideal weight. These charts DO take your age into account and so they already allow a little extra weight, so don't overdo this. But do not aim for the lower part of "normal" this is too much weight loss.

But there are many people, and I agree with their outlook in general, who say that if someone WANTS to be overweight then we should not class them as having a problem. If they are overweight and healthy, then that is up to them, but if someone is overweight and it is clearly affecting their health then I would hope that they find the willpower, or even just the desire to lose a few pounds.

Whatever you select as your ideal weight, I hope that you find that this diet will help you to achieve it, and I honestly believe that it will if you follow the basic guidelines.

I hope that you will soon HAVE to read the section on what to do when you reach your target weight, that will be a great day for you (and for me, if I know that I have been able to help you).

Diet for health reasons

My one fear is that this diet may trigger a health problem such as anorexia or bulimia; it is this fear that has made me think long and hard before deciding to write this book. I don't want anyone to be harmed by anything in this book, so please do not use this diet if you are already at a "normal" weight for your size and age.

Let me explain it in the following way;

You can probably take one look at someone and instantly decide if they look good, ugly, overweight, skinny, etc. etc. BUT you can look at yourself in a mirror for AGES and not really know how to judge yourself.

For example I KNOW that I am not handsome, but this is not by looking at myself in a mirror, it is based on experiences throughout my life. If I look in the mirror, all I see is ME! I don't see a stranger, I see the same old me that I have seen for years. I don't see any subtle changes and I have seen myself every day and so I cannot judge myself, I looked like this yesterday and the day before and so on. Even though I may have changed over time I could not perceive those changes because they happened gradually and I see myself every day.

This means that we cannot really judge our own appearance; yes we can tell if we look good in some clothes that we are wearing, but we cannot really judge ourselves properly.

So when it comes to our shape and physical appearance we HAVE to rely on others to judge us, but even then this is often not an honest or correct opinion. The "bullies" of this world believe that the only way for them to get ahead is to push other people down, so they will always tell you that you are ugly, fat, or whatever. It can therefore be very hard to obtain a true judgement of what you are and what you look like.

So PLEASE be very careful about your weight; believe the charts that show your BMI, if you are at the bottom of the "normal" range then you are NOT overweight regardless of your own (inaccurate) opinion of how you look.

If your appearance is VERY important to you it can be easy to go too far and push yourself further than necessary. You may feel that you are fat but you might not have noticed the gradual differences due to your losing weight on your diet. So this can lead to you having an "internal picture" of yourself that does not match reality.

When it comes to weight you DO have an independent view on whether you are overweight or not, this is the BMI chart again. You do not need to ask someone if you are overweight, this chart will give you a very clear indication, if it indicates that your weight is normal then it IS normal, no matter what picture you have in your head of how you look. (A BMI chart is available at www. thebirchalldiet.com)

So PLEASE do not use this or any other diet if you are already at the healthy weight that you should be, according to the BMI chart.

ONLY diet if your weight is causing you health problems, this includes if you are marginally overweight according to the BMI chart and just feel bad about yourself. But STOP when you reach the middle of your range.

If you are not dieting for health reasons or if you are only dieting because you want to be skinny, then PLEASE do not diet at all.

WHAT MAKES OUR WEIGHT INCREASE?

Please forgive me for oversimplifying this but the ONLY way that your weight increases is by the weight of the food that you eat or drink.

There are no magical occurrences, no mysteries, it is plain and simple; if you eat something weighing 2 pounds your weight will increase by two pounds, no more and no less. It makes no difference WHAT you eat, the result is the same.

Eat two pounds of sugar, two pounds (in weight) of water, two pounds of fat, two pounds of steak etc. etc. it makes no difference they will ALL make your weight increase by two pounds.

This is exactly why you should avoid diet foods and diet drinks etc. (unless you enjoy them that is). They all add weight, just like the non-diet version of that food or drink. They are not magical or mysterious, the difference is that the diet foods contain little or no fuel and so can be expelled quite quickly and easily. Non-diet versions will contain some fuel but your body NEEDS fuel so it is OK to use non-diet versions as long as you are not having too much. If the diet versions contain no fuel then why bother having them? Could it be that you see this as a way of holding off the hunger? In which case we have already covered why we actually NEED to experience the hunger sensation, to lose weight.

If you think about it, a can of diet drink weighs exactly the same as a can of non-diet drink. The difference is how well your body can use what you have eaten or drunk and how much of it is retained. The sugar in non-diet drinks does not do anything that breaks the basic laws of science it cannot increase your weight by more than its own weight. So it is just that your body can burn that sugar instead of your reserves of fat and so it delays your weight loss slightly.

One way to reduce your weight is to reduce the weight of the food that you are eating (again apologies for stating the obvious but this whole diet is based on understanding some of the basics that we take for granted). Smaller portions mean less weight and if those smaller portions are high grade fuels then your body can survive on a smaller weight of food just as well as it can on a larger weight of low grade fuel.

Keep the weight down of what you are eating and you will keep your own weight down. Eating lighter portions of "normal" foods results in less weight on the scales.

The next section covers how we LOSE weight (again VERY basic) and between the two we can learn to control our weight and lose it as and when we want to.

WHAT MAKES OUR WEIGHT DECREASE?

Again, this is VERY basic, there is no mystery involved. You do not simply "burn off" weight. The only way your weight decreases is when you visit the toilet or when you perspire (at least the only significant way). I am not including the weight you lose when you breath out moisture, trim your nails or when you get a hair cut, sneeze, pick your nose, shed skin, cut your finger off etc.!

Again, we have to consider the laws of science; weight (mass) does not just disappear. So we lose weight mainly though urine and the "other toilet thing". But of these two we need to focus on urine.

We urinate several times a day (and when we get a little older, we urinate several times a night too!). This is where MOST of our weight loss occurs and so we need to use this to our advantage. We need to try to eat foods that are high in liquid content so that our body can get rid of that weight quickly. That is why our "squashable / dilutable" guide for the food we eat, is important. It is easy to get rid of this type of food, mostly through urine, meat and other foods that are not "squashable / dilutable" has to wait until we visit the toilet for "the other thing".

When I say "Squashable / Dilutable" I do not mean that you have to eat squashed or diluted foods. I am just suggesting that you focus on foods that COULD be squashed easily (by reasonably light pressure from a fork) or foods that are affected by water (they break down into pieces or are thinned out by it). I am not for one minute saying that you should eat liquidised foods. It is vitally important that you enjoy the food that you do eat. I for one would not eat liquidised foods apart from a nice wholesome soup.

Overnight we often lose anything up to a couple of pounds of weight, just by sleeping and urinating the next morning. A larger than usual part of this can be perspiration; you would be surprised how much we lose. I have seen demonstrations where a couple were locked into a completely dry airtight room overnight (with enough oxygen to breathe of course!), then the following morning special extractors were used to recover the fluids they lost and there were PINTS of the stuff (not a pleasant sight but remarkable all the same). So keep nice and warm overnight (not too warm of course, just warm enough to be comfortable) this is one of the easiest ways to lose a tiny amount of weight without doing anything!!!

If you exercise to lose weight, try weighing yourself before and then after the exercise with accurate scales. The only weight loss you will see at that point will be totally due to perspiration. You will not have magically burnt off any weight, but what will happen is that your body will have used some of the fat reserves and converted this to energy and in doing so will have produced urine. Urinating after the exercise is how the weight is lost, it does not just disappear. Also have you ever noticed that after a lot of exercise your urine may be darker or seem stronger? This is because this is affected by the residue created when your fat is converted during exercise.

If you drink lots of water while you are exercising (as you should, to replace the fluids lost via perspiration) the net effect may be no weight loss at all, but soon after you will urinate and probably more than usual and then you lose the weight. You also have to consider that some of the fat may have been converted to muscle due to the exercise and muscle is heavier than fat and so the actual weight loss due to exercise may well be less than you had hoped. I always maintain that you should exercise to keep fit and NOT to lose weight.

So stop thinking that you burn off weight, you only really lose any weight down the toilet or from perspiration.

WHAT MAKES US GAIN WEIGHT OVER TIME?

Quite simply your weight will increase over time if you are putting in more food than you are getting rid of. I know that this sounds like an over-simplification (again) but it isn't. Many people concentrate on calories, points etc. and these <u>may</u> have an effect, but the actual weight gain is not relevant to the calories or points, it is simply that you have eaten more than you have despatched down the toilet.

So what can make us retain some of the food we have eaten? In truth the only way that your body will retain this weight is by it being stored as fat reserves or possibly as muscle. If you have eaten more fuel than you body needs to burn, the excess (or at least a lot of it) will be stored for use later, as fat reserves. If you are exercising a lot, then some of it will also be stored as muscle tissue.

If our weight increases simply because we are retaining some of the food we eat as fat or muscle, then we can use this knowledge to control how much we retain. In short, we need to eat foods that do not stay around in our stomach for long, but more importantly we need to eat ONLY enough of whatever it is we are eating, to give us the energy we need to "get by". If we eat more fuel than we need, our body will store this as fat reserves and so we will be outputting less than we input.

So we gain weight by eating more fuel than we need. Note that I say fuel rather than food; this is because this totally depends on <u>what</u> food we are eating. It does not matter what food we eat when it comes to JUST weight control (leaving aside healthy eating for a moment), the most important thing is to eat the right amount of fuel and the amount of fuel in your food varies depending on what you are eating.

To eat a set amount of fuel means different volumes of foods depending on what we are eating. If we are eating low calorie or diet foods we will have to eat far more in volume to get the same amount of fuel from non diet, "normal" foods. The one thing that we must NOT do is to eat a high volume of non diet, "normal" foods, because these are rich in fuel. This is why many diets persuade you to eat foods that contain less fuel; the theory is that you are eating less fuel because you are eating food with less fuel in it. But by doing this you often eat more in volume for the same fuel rating?

 If you were to focus on eating the right amount of fuel instead of using diet foods then you can control this even more easily. I prefer to eat normal foods in less volume and get exactly the same fuel as I would from a higher volume of diet foods.

What makes us lose weight over time?

I would imagine that you can guess what I am going to say here? It is pretty basic; you lose weight over time by eating LESS food than you get rid of.

But it is NOT just a question of volume of food; you have to eat less fuel than your body needs so that it has to burn off the excess fat that it has stored in reserve. To do this you have to eat little and often and stop "stocking up" on food at meal times (this just ADDS to the very reserves that we are trying to get rid of)

Eat just enough fuel to get you to the next snack allow yourself to feel slightly hungry for a while and give your body chance to burn off the excess fat it has stored.

This is the basis of this diet, eating little and often, eating foods that can be processed very quickly and allowing your body to burn off the excess fat.

By eating foods that are high in water / liquid content you can get rid of the food very quickly via urinating. Eat foods that are high in fuel and low in volume / weight (diet foods are LOW in fuel and High in volume / weight.).

I will not cover the whole diet in this chapter, I will cover this in a different chapter, but you have to aim to eat less FUEL than you need (but still enough to survive and stay healthy).

Stephen Birchall

WHAT IS SO DIFFERENT ABOUT THIS DIET?

The major difference about this diet is that other diets try to give you lots of different ways to suppress your hunger. They suggest diet drinks / foods, low calorie snacks, even water, as a means to stop you feeling hungry while you are dieting. This diet sees the hunger sensation as a positive one to be encouraged, the hunger sensation means that you are burning up (converting) the excess fat that your body has stored.

I believe that if you mask the hunger sensation you are actually slowing down the process of weight loss. So while you are on this diet you should be AIMING to feel slightly hungry for at least part of the day, the longer you can experience the hunger the better but in NO WAY must you starve yourself, this is totally unnecessary and can cause serious problems. Just let yourself feel peckish and when this becomes too uncomfortable, eat something with fuel in it.

Diet foods are not only unnecessary on this diet, they should be avoided! You should be having a lower VOLUME of food that has the same "fuel rating" instead of a large volume of "low fuel" food. This allows your stomach to get used to smaller portions and for it to shrink down in size naturally over time.

Many other diets suggest eating "little and often" as a guide, but this really is a mainstay in this diet, even to the extent of replacing your regular meals with snacks (so you can diet AND still have the social pleasure of group meals). This is covered in later chapters in detail.

No foods are banned on this diet, meats and chicken etc. are to be avoided but they are certainly not banned. You MUST be able to enjoy your food or you will never stick to a diet.

Exercise is NOT part of this diet, although you should have regular exercise for HEALTH reasons.

Most importantly, there are no charts, no points systems, no need to read labels (again apart from health reasons); it is almost like you can diet without being on a diet!

Another important difference with this diet is that it explains the logic behind all of the recommendations and allows YOU to be the expert when it comes to YOUR body. There are no lists of do's and don'ts that make no sense, there are no unexplained theories such as how many points are in a specific food, or how many calories YOUR body needs.

In all I would like to think that this is a completely different way of thinking about dieting. Not only does it make YOU the expert but it also relies on your body's amazing abilities to control its own weight.

THE HUNGER SENSATION

This is the most "Radical" part of this diet and I hope that you can use this to your advantage.

We all THINK that we know what we mean when we say that we are "hungry" and we are ALMOST correct. This hunger sensation IS a signal to tell us to eat, BUT, and it is a big BUT (no pun intended), it is slightly more than that.

As I have said already on several occasions, your body is an amazing thing, it can do so much and we probably know more about the universe than we do about the abilities of our own mind and body. If you can believe this, and I hope that you can, then you can perhaps believe that your body can issue very complex signals and perhaps in this case it is more refined than to simply have a hunger signal.

One way to understand what I am saying is when you feel hungry you don't simply feel hungry, you feel like very specific foods. Sometimes you feel hungry for something sweet (especially juts after a meal, that is why we like to have a desert course if we can), sometimes we feel hungry for something salty or savoury (often to balance out an excess of liquid that we have consumed, often a reason for the amount of crisps, peanuts etc, sold in bars). Our body is not just sending signals for food, it is trying to balance the complex chemicals that we need to survive and grow. So we need to treat our "hunger sensation" with more respect and use it in our diet, not only to lose weight but to also ensure that we are eating the correct foods to enable us to have a balanced diet.

I also think that there are two different signals that we class as being one "hunger" signal. I believe that the main signal we get is NOT telling us to eat something it is merely a signal that warns us that we are starting to consume our reserves of fat (which in itself would normally be an indicator that we should be eating something). The difference is quite subtle but VERY important. If the signal is merely telling us that your body is now consuming your reserves, then this is exactly what we want to experience if we want to lose weight.

Think about it this way, if our body normally uses the fuel in our stomach to power it, if we started to take fuel from our reserve fat (mainly around our belly) instead we would surely notice a different sensation?? This is what I believe we incorrectly class as the hunger sensation, we are actually feeling our fat reserves being converted..

So if we realise that this sensation that we call hunger could be the sensation we feel when our body is consuming the excess fat it has stored, then we can use this to our advantage. Whenever we feel this sensation it is like having an instant indication that we are losing weight at that exact moment. We can therefore know when we are losing weight and choose just how long we want to carry on for.

Other diets that tell you to drink water, or a diet food / drink of some kind to mask this sensation could be stopping you from burning up the very fat that you are trying to get rid of. This COULD help to explain why so many of the other diets fail.

You should think of this hunger sensation as a POSITIVE signal and try to put up with the mild discomfort for a short while, instead of grabbing something to get rid of it as soon as it starts. It is important to realise that I am not saying that you should starve yourself, this simply would not work, not only would you make yourself ill but you would never be able to continue such a diet for long.

So use this sensation to enable you to control your own weight, if you are not feeling hungry then you are simply not losing weight (or at least not losing much weight). Make sure that you allow yourself to feel this sensation before you decide to eat something else. This way you can stop yourself from adding MORE fat reserves, your body will take the main part of its fuel from your reserves instead of from your stomach.

Do we need meals at all?

This may seem like a stupid question, surely the answer is "of course we need meals, we are human, and humans eat meals"? I know this may sound radical but I would like to challenge this. Perhaps we USED TO have to eat meals and perhaps things have changed but we have yet to realise it?

I always like to break things down to the basics and there is so much going on in the modern world that it is often not easy to determine what is actually happening. So I would like to look at this whole concept of meals from a very different viewpoint. Let's just go back in time to the era when we all lived in caves and life was much harder but also much more basic.

Food was available, but only after a lot of effort to obtain it. Either a long walk to find fruits and vegetable etc. (there were no farms then) or tracking and capturing animals. All of this took a LOT of time, energy and effort and there would be long gaps in between where there was no food at all. So when we did have food, we gorged on it and ate as much of it as we could possibly fit in our stomach before the animal rotted and became inedible (no fridges then either!). We then had to use a lot of energy to track down the next "meal" and the gap sometimes meant that we had to rely on the fat reserves that our body had stored from the last huge meal we ate. This was therefore the only option available, there is no way that we could snack we did not have access to any foods "on tap". So we lived on a cycle of overeating, starving, hunting, starving, overeating etc. This was not exactly the same as sitting down to breakfast, lunch, dinner etc. but it was certainly not eating "little and often" either.

As we progressed over time, we developed farming and methods of storing foods, but even then there was no concept of snacks (the nearest we got to this was walking past a tree at the right time of year and noticing berries etc.). So we had to eat when the food was available and then wait until the next food was available. As we progressed and food became more readily available due to farming etc. this became more and more regimented and we developed meal times.

One of the main reasons that these mealtimes became regular and divided throughout the day was due to the fact that we had to cook and prepare our food. This had to be at set times throughout the day so that the effort in preparing the food was made more manageable. Cooking was such a task then that you would not want to have to do it several times a day. So meals were prepared for breakfast (when everyone was together before they left for work, school etc.), Lunch (when the breakfast had "worn off" and most people had to top up again in the middle of the day to get them through to the last meal at dinner (when everyone was back from work, school etc.).

So meals developed from convenience and the tools and skills that were available. The problem is that we have moved on yet again and we have not yet changed our habits to match. How many times have you heard experts telling us that we are all getting more and more overweight and we are, on average, more overweight now than we have ever been? I believe that there is a reason for this and that reason is SNACKS! The very thing I have been recommending in this diet.

I believe that for the first time in human history we now have the ability to snack all day long on wholesome (and some not so wholesome) foods. BUT, and it is a BIG BUT (another BIG BUT), the thing that we are getting wrong is that we eat our meals and then snack all day AS WELL !!!

We have all been brought up to eat a meal at mealtimes and have even been told not to eat much between meals. This WAS very sound advice, but the problem is that now if we feel hungry between meals there is always something to hand. The hunger sensation is uncomfortable and so if we CAN stop it we WILL. This means that we NEVER allow ourselves to feel hungry and so effectively we never allow our body to consume the reserves that it has built up, hence we never lose weight.

So I believe that we are living in VERY different times now and so I would like to challenge our approach to how often and when we eat.

Is it possible that we no longer need to eat meals at all? It sounds very radical and I am not expecting you to give up your meals, but let's just look at it from a different angle. If food is our source of fuel, then by overfilling our "fuel tank" (our stomach) we are forcing our bodies to store the extra fuel as fat. It would surely be far better to ensure that we continue to take in fuel at small regular intervals as and when we use it, so that we never overfill the tank and yet make sure that we never run out of fuel either?

Perhaps this only appears radical because we come from a generation that HAD to rely on meals for their fuel. We simply didn't have easy access to decent foods upon demand. Even as recent as 100 years ago, or less, the option of snacking was not really available. There were no fridges, no packets of crisps, sweets were very rare, cooking was not as simple as it is now (no microwave ovens, pot noodles etc.) etc. etc. and so you HAD to eat a large meal to keep you going to the next meal.

Is it really radical? Or is it just that we can change our habits to match our environment, and this has changed dramatically in recent years and we have not yet adapted to it.

In fact this could be the cause of many people becoming overweight, now we can have our meals AND snack all day. You can cut out the snacks (or have low cal / diet snacks) and just have the meals, but then you will have to store the extra food that we eat at mealtimes, as fat for reserves. So why not cut out (or more sensibly, cut down on) the meals and eat little and often throughout the day.

Meals can be important socially and so the whole family / friends can still sit together, but you don't HAVE to go for the full-on three course meal or even eat such a large meal that you feel full (or worse still, bloated).

Why not try a one or two course meal instead with slightly smaller portions and with something that matches the guidelines of this diet (squashable / dilutable foods).

This is the first era EVER in the history of humankind, where it is easy to maintain a good healthy food supply throughout the day, eating on demand, rather than having to wait until meal times and gorge ourselves to give us enough reserves to get us through to the next meal and so on. Now we have snacks of all types and sizes and so we do not need to fill the tank each time, we can snack throughout the day and not build up huge reserves.

So why not try changing and not have a full meal, just have a large snack at meal times instead, but remember that it is also important to make your diet less like torture and so still have the meals and visits to the restaurant as and when you want to, they are very important, but understand how this affects you and accept that this will delay your weight loss for a few days, it is not the end of the world, there are no rigid rules in this diet.

So, as radical as it may have sounded, I hope that you can see that we should at least be able to challenge the concept that we have to stuff ourselves at mealtimes to get us through to the next meal. Often people talk about "little and often" as being a good way to eat, I couldn't agree more and I hope that I have perhaps explained the reasons why this is a good approach and one that I feel is essential if you are trying to lose weight.

HAVE A SNACK AT MEALTIME

This is one of the biggest changes you can make to your diet and there are MANY benefits, so please do give it a try.

As we have already explained, it is really good for you to eat "little and often", this applies at meal times in particular. Instead of having a full meal with all of the courses / extras, try to have a snack (perhaps a slightly larger snack).

As covered in the section / chapter "Do we need meals at all?" we are now in a period in time where we do not HAVE to eat a full meal to tide us over until we can eat again. We can snack all day if we want to, so we do not have to "stock up" on food at meal times. Any excess food will just add more fat at a time that we are trying to lose it.

You simply do not have to have a large plateful of food anymore. Just have a smaller portion (small enough to just take the edge off your hunger), you can always have a snack later when you want to stop the hunger sensation.

By never eating enough food to fill your stomach, you cannot build up more fat reserves, so never eat enough to make you feel full (unless you are treating yourself and having a meal out or with friends).

In many cases it is important for the family to get together at meal times, IN NO WAY am I suggesting that you stop this, you can still sit down for meals with the family but just have LESS.

Remember that you need fuel to survive; excess fuel will be stored in reserve as fat, so just eat enough to get you to the next snack, instead of filling your tank at each mealtime.

Meals out with loved ones (or even your Spouse!), or meals with friends are important social occasions, so these are not banned in this diet, in fact they are actively encouraged. A large meal will slow down your weight loss for a few days and that is not the end of the world. But if you decline such meals or go for the "I am on a diet, I am different" meal selections, then you will quickly stop dieting.

No pain, no gain is an overused saying but it does apply to ANY diet. But that pain must be bearable and the benefits of the diet must outweigh that pain.

So at mealtimes try leaving out some of the "extras" and just have the main part of the meal, or simply reduce the size of the meal to just enough to take the edge off your hunger. If you can eat a meal (large snack) and come away from the table still feeling "peckish" then this is perfect. You have given your body the fuel it needs and yet have not eaten enough to add any more reserve fuel.

As for what you should eat at meal times, the same guideline applies, have something "squashable / dilutable" and avoid meat, chicken or any other similar food (Tuna is fine but a tuna steak is VERY similar to meat in that it is so solid that it will take a long time for your body to break it down and digest it). If you are not sure, have a look at the section later in the book that discusses the various food types and how they will affect your diet. But you will not go far wrong if you follow the guideline.

Avoid a meal or snack just before bedtime, have something at least an hour or so before you go to bed and try to stick to a snack that is very liquid, or even just a drink. The food you eat just before you go to bed will be available for your body to fully digest for many hours while you sleep, so try to go to bed with just a little food in your stomach (you can burn off a reasonable amount of weight while you sleep and you will not notice your hunger sensations even when you wake (until some time later).

LITTLE AND OFTEN

We have already covered this in other sections but it is very important.

You must realise exactly what we mean by this "over-used" saying, you should try to never totally fill your stomach at any time, even at meal times.

Snacks are readily available these days and most people can snack throughout the day (even if this is just by keeping a few biscuits or sweets in your pocket / purse).

We are trying to get rid of our fat that our body has stored for later use, so not only do we have to make sure that we consume this fat, but we must try to avoid adding any more.

By eating small portions of food at mealtimes you will need to snack often. The smaller portions will not get you from one mealtime to another, so snacking has to become part of your daily routine.

Many people see snacking as something to be avoided on a diet but this is only true if you are eating "normal" meals AND snacking. What we need to do is to switch to snacking ONLY.

When you start to feel hungry or peckish, remember that this is a clear indication that you are losing weight, so do not simply try to stop the hunger sensation as soon as it starts. Drinking water or having something "diet" may SEEM to be the thing to do, but this just stops you from feeling hungry and so stops you from losing weight (remember what the "hunger sensation" really is, it is just your body consuming the reserve fat it has stored, it is NOT just a hunger signal).

Let yourself feel hungry for a short while (do NOT let yourself starve to the point of feeling tired, ill or having dizzy spells etc. you simply don't need to starve yourself on this diet). When you have decided that you have felt hungry for a while and you now have to eat something, do NOT eat something diet or low calorie etc. your body has sent clear signals that it needs some fuel, give it some proper fuel. Eat something that your body is clearly indicating that it needs. You will find that you are hungry for specific foods or drinks; you might feel like something sweet or something salty etc. Listen to your body and eat what you feel like. BUT this is PROPER food and so be careful about the amount of food that you are eating. Eat just enough to ease your hunger, if you still feel hungry a few minutes later (30 minutes at least) then have some more of whatever you feel like now (it may be something different now).

Whatever you do, do not just eat something else, just because you "normally eat X at this time of day". Eat what you body is asking for or you may find that you have eaten something else and your body is still demanding the food it originally wanted as well as the food you just ate.

Keep trying to eat small volumes of "normal" foods throughout the day and don't have "peaks" and "troughs". This way you will not only lose weight, but you will also educate, or reduce your stomach to cope with the new volumes of foods you are now eating.

Not only will you reduce your weight AND your stomach, but you will almost certainly reduce the amount of money you spend on food each week and even reduce the size of your food larder. In all a "Win, Win, Win" situation.

Eating slowly

Many people will tell you that eating your food slowly is important if you are on a diet and in most cases they are absolutely correct. But there are exceptions where it does not really make any difference at all.

Firstly why does it help to eat slowly rather than quickly? The reason for this is the time it takes for your body to realise that you have eaten the food.

Consider the example where you are hungry and you feel like some chocolate and so you eat a single square of chocolate (which is ok on this diet). By the time you have finished that square of chocolate you are still craving some more chocolate and so you have another square, and so on and so on. Your body takes time to process the chocolate and extract the goodness that it craved from that chocolate, this can be several minutes. Imagine the process that it goes through, it has to reach your stomach first, and then it has to be dissolved and the ingredients broken down and absorbed. Then the "message" has to be sent to your brain to indicate that your body now has what it needed. In the time this has taken you could have eaten far more than was needed. So in this case eating slowly works very well, in fact if it was something like chocolate I would eat a square or two and then wait ten minutes, if I still felt like I wanted some more chocolate I would have another piece.

Where eating slowly has little or no effect is when you fully intended to eat everything anyway. So if you have a plate of food in front of you and you intend eating every bit of it, then eating slowly is not going to make much difference. It will still make SOME difference but not a lot; it will possibly help in that you may not feel like a desert if your body has had time to digest the food you have just eaten. But the major benefit of eating slowly is when you use it to reduce the amount that you are eating.

A side benefit to eating slowly is that you get longer to enjoy the flavours of the food and this could help satisfy you more easily. If you used to eat a large portion of your favourite food because you liked to savour the flavour for a long time, if you are having a smaller portion now, eating it slowly means that you can savour the flavour for just as long as before and still have less. Rushing your food may result in little or no pleasure for you and so you may feel that you need some more, so take your time and enjoy the flavour (you will also find that your food tastes better when you are on this diet and so you could get even MORE enjoyment from your food, even with smaller portions).

So my suggestion is to eat everything a little slower than you normally would, to give your body time to process the food and determine if more is needed. But to gain major benefits, do this in conjunction with a decision that you do not have to eat everything that is on the plate (or the whole bar or bag of crisps or whatever you are eating).

Stephen Birchall

Finishing your food

You must remember that you never have to finish your food completely; this includes snacks as well as meals.

I am sure that you have been told time and time again that wasting food is bad, "think of all of the starving children in the world....." etc. However true the sentiment is, it is very important when dieting to never eat too much, especially with this particular diet. We must avoid over eating of any amount especially at "meal times".

Feeling compelled to clear your plate of food or finish the whole bar of chocolate WILL harm your weight loss. The last couple of mouthfuls on the plate, or the last few squares of chocolate will go straight back into your "reserve fat" and hold up your weight loss. Always stop when you have had enough no matter how much (or how little) is left.

If you can manage to finish eating and still feel peckish then that is perfect, don't eat until you feel full or that will mean that you have enough food to enable your body to store some for later and that weight takes effort to remove it.

If you have every intention of eating every mouthful of the food then still eat slowly even though it will not directly help you eat less (you are going to eat it all anyway). This will allow you to enjoy the food more, even if it is a smaller portion.

Let's use the example of where you are going out for a special meal, or a meal with friends. You really want to enjoy your meal and you feel like having the steak (or whatever your favourite meal is. There is absolutely no need to miss out, have your choice but if there is an option of a smaller portion then go for that.

So you have your meal in front of you and it is smaller than you really wanted, this is where eating slowly pays dividends. If you would have gone for a larger portion, it would have taken longer to eat and you would have been able to enjoy your favourite treat for longer. By eating slowly, you can savour each mouthful for longer and STILL eat a smaller portion.

The other hidden bonus on this diet is that you will soon discover that by putting up with the hunger sensation for a while throughout the day you will enjoy the flavour and sensation of your food a LOT more than you ever used to. So a smaller portion of your favourite food, eaten slowly, can mean that you can probably enjoy it more than usual, finish you meal and still be controlling your weight.

I really do like this diet, it works and yet I can still thoroughly enjoy eating!!!!!!!!

SETTING A TARGET WEIGHT

Setting the correct target weight is important; please don't just pick a target without thinking it through.

If you pick a target that is going to be very difficult to achieve then you may do extremely well on your diet but leave yourself feeling as if you have somehow failed because you did not reach your target. Even though this "failure" is more likely to be due to the target being too aggressive, it could still feel like a failure and it shouldn't do. For a diet to work you need to feel as if you are in control, if you feel that you are in control then you can handle the inevitable "blips" where your weight may suddenly go up a bit. To feel in control you have to set sensible targets that you should be able to hit and then, if you want set new targets and so on until you are at the ideal weight for your size.

It is much less of a problem if you set a relatively easy target to hit, because if you manage to achieve that target then there is nothing stopping you from setting a new one.

But the main thing to remember is that the diet should be aimed at getting you to a healthy weight, it should not be just about body shape or a weight that you THINK is good for you. There are plenty of charts around giving you the ideal BMI and these all give you a range that is considered to be appropriate to your height. I recommend that you use these recommendations when considering your ultimate target weight.

The first target weight that you set should be quite a modest loss, we need to have a positive experience and build on that. I cannot recommend how many pounds you should aim for at first because this obviously depends on how overweight you are. But aim for your first target weight to be more than your ideal weight so that you can see what happens. You may find that the weight drops off quicker than you thought (hopefully) and this could give you a really positive experience. But if your weight loss is initially a bit slower than you hoped you still have a target that you can achieve.

Before you start the diet (if it is not too late), work out the recommended BMI for your height and set an ultimate target that is the equivalent of the high end of the "normal" BMI . This should be the MAXIMUM that you want to lose; don't try to hit the lower range of the recommended BMI. I always maintain that to be healthy you have to have some reserves of fat; you never know when you might need them. Aiming for too high a target is better than aiming too low, so perhaps set a target weight that you would like to hit within X weeks and then review it at that time.

I set myself a target of 7lbs initially but hit this so quickly that I changed it to 10lbs. Then when I hit that target I decided to stay at that weight for a while because I REALLY did not think that I could ever get to my "ideal" weight according to the BMI charts. To achieve that would have meant a total loss of 32 lbs (from 16 stone 4lbs to 14 stone) and before I tried my new diet I was pretty sure that this would be impossible for me. But after stabilising my weight for a week or so (at my initial target weight) I found it so easy to lose a few more pounds and so I decided to "go for gold" and get to the top band of a "normal" BMI instead of being in the middle to high band of "overweight". I reached my absolute target weight without much fuss and have been able to keep it at this level, even though I eat out a lot.

So set a small target at first to see how you get on with this new diet and modify that target based on how successful it is for you. Hopefully you will soon be setting (and hitting) your ultimate target of a good healthy weight.

WHAT TO DO WHEN YOU REACH YOUR TARGET WEIGHT

If you need to read this part of the book, then congratulations, you must be nearing or have achieved your target weight.

Even if this is just the fact that you have reached your initial target weight and you plan on continuing to a new (ultimate?) target weight, you still need to pause and consider what to do next. It is important to remember that most diets will help you lose weight, but this is a waste of time if you just put it all (and more?) back on again.

So do make sure that you understand what has happened and what you now need to do.

If you have lost a reasonable amount of weight on this diet (and there is no reason why you shouldn't have) then it is vital to realise HOW this worked for you. I would suggest that you re-read some of the main sections again and see if you can agree with how and why you were able to do this. The reason is that once you hit your target weight you need to switch more to "weight control" than "weight loss". This diet will work best if you are completely in control and can lose, retain or even gain weight as and when you want to. To achieve this you need to understand how it has worked for you and which elements of the diet were most beneficial.

Some people do not follow a diet to the letter, this is fine, but if it has worked then it is important to know which parts of it worked best for you. For some people, the "hunger sensation" is the key and is responsible for most of the weight loss, for others it could be the "squashable / dilutable" guide that has helped the most. Some may have benefited most from the regular weigh-ins and so on.

Hopefully you will have followed most of the guidelines and found the whole of the diet useful, but whatever worked for you, the most important thing is that it DID work and so you need to build on this.

If you have reached an early target and need to continue through to another target, just continue as you are but see if there are any suggestions that you may have not been following. It might also help if you spend a few days just trying to stabilise your weight first, before you press on to the next target. This will ensure that you feel in control of your weight as well as giving you chance to ease off a little for a short while, after all, we want you to be able to stick with the diet, long term and not for just one big "hit" that could lead to you putting the weight back on.

If you have reached your ultimate target and are now happy with your weight, then this is fantastic, you have made it. Find some photographs of the "old" you and remind yourself of just how much you have achieved. Use this as a reminder if you ever see the pounds piling on again.

The most important thing now is to make sure that you do not put the weight back on, but it is also as important to be careful that you do not continue to lose weight and become under-weight. This diet can be so successful that you MAY find that the weight continues to fall after you have reached your target. If this happens, simply increase your portion size slightly and avoid the hunger sensation for a while.

To maintain a steady weight you should continue with exactly the same process as you did when you were losing weight, but now you must not leave yourself feeling the "hunger sensation" for long. When this hits, just eat something with lots of energy in it to keep the hunger off for a while. Continue snacking and eating little and often, but ensure that your portions are large enough to ease the hunger sensation without ever feeling full.

Pay close attention to the scales, still weigh yourself at least every morning and watch out for any signs of the weight returning. You do not need to react to every tiny movement, if you have put on one pound then just avoid putting on another pound, don't immediately try and lose it. But you should find that you are in complete control now and you can lose any extra weight as and when you want to by adjusting how long you allow yourself to feel hungry.

You may need to keep adjusting things for a few weeks while your weight stabilises, but the regular weigh-ins should help. You also need to remember how difficult it was to lose weight initially and so watch those scales very carefully and act on any weight gains if they seem to be setting in.

But during this diet your basic volume of food should have reduced considerably and this will lead to your stomach capacity reducing. This in itself will help you to keep the pounds off and so you probably will not have to do much at all, you will probably find that your new approach to eating will be enough, after all we are using the ability that our body has built-in to regulate its own weight and so it should be able to look after itself (as long as we "listen to" and understand the messages we get from it.)

As time goes by you can reduce the weigh-ins to every other morning, but try to keep weighing yourself at least three times a week until you can be sure that your weight has stabilised.

I would be very grateful if you could let me know of your success, please feel free to post your messages to the forum at www. thebirchalldiet.com. I am hoping that hearing your success story may spur on other people who also want to lose weight. Remember how you felt before and after the diet? It would be fantastic if you can help someone else experience this great feeling of achievement.

Why do some diets just not work for me?

Most diets focus on ensuring that you eat less, either in calories, in points, in volume or in the type of food that you eat. There is nothing wrong in that of course, but many diets miss one important fact. We are all different and even people with the same body shape and size are very different in the way that food affects them. How many times have you heard someone say, "I just have to LOOK at a chocolate bar and I put 2 lbs on, yet she (he) seems to be able to eat chocolate all day". Food affects different people in different ways, so there is no real formula that can be ideal for everyone.

What would work is if the "expert" could create a diet specifically for YOU and monitor everything that you eat and tell you what to eat and when. But this is just not going to happen, or is it???

What if there was an expert that knew exactly when you had had enough food, when you need to eat something very specific, what to eat next, exactly when you are losing weight minute by minute? THERE IS SUCH AN EXPERT ----- YOU !!!!!!! (or at least your body is the expert).

We all have an inbuilt mechanism that can control our weight, our own body sends out signals when it is time to eat, it indicates WHAT to eat and also indicates when you have had enough. So you need to listen to THIS expert and not the others.

In addition to this, your body will need different foods and volumes depending on what you have been doing. You will need a different amount of calories, points, carbs, fat, etc. etc. depending on how active you have been. Spend all day sitting in an office and your body will need a certain amount and type of food to match. Spend the day gardening, or exercising and your needs will be different. But the important thing is HOW different? No expert can tell you this, therefore most diets will not adapt to your differing requirements. That is often the reason why diets don't work for some people.

To me though, most diets fail for one main reason, they tell you how to lose weight and NOT feel hungry. They recommend drinking water to ease your hunger, or have a diet yoghurt, have some muesli for breakfast (or other "slow release" food).

I hope that you have already agreed with my thoughts on the "hunger sensation" and how this is a clear indication that your body is burning up some excess fat that it has stored? If you do agree with this, or at least that it is POSSIBLE, then you can now see why these other diets sometimes fail. If they tell you ways to diet without feeling hungry, then you are dieting without feeling the sensation of your body burning up the fat. Does this mean that they do not believe in the "no pain, no gain" principle? I do, I really believe that to lose this extra weight we need to go against this one signal that our body is sending out and endure the slight discomfort for a short while at least. If we do not experience this then all we are doing is reducing the effect of whatever diet we are on.

So if you have tried diets that help you hide the hunger, this might be the reason why they did not work for you.

Some people simply do not like using charts, points, counting calories etc. It can be very cumbersome and time consuming. It is certainly something that you do not want to have to do when eating out, there is nothing like a diet fanatics ranting about how many points there are in a salad, to kill the conversation at a special meal with friends or family. So perhaps the diets that force you to read labels and calculate points are simply not for you. Shopping can be a real pain if you have to read the fine print of every label just so that you can tell how "bad" it is for your diet.

Diets that mean separate foods for me and "normal" foods for everyone else in the family do not work for me either. Shopping is enough of a chore already let's not make it any worse than it has to be.

I always believe that there is NO POINT in eating any food that has no points in it anyway (apart from the occasion portion for the vitamins etc. So these diets certainly do not work for me!)

What also happens on some diets is that they are persuading you to eat foods that you don't actually feel like eating. Your body might be sending out signals that you need something sweet, but sugar may be banned on the diet and so you have something else instead. But your body needed that sugar (or whatever it was craving), so it will keep on prompting you to eat it sooner or later and the chances are that you will give in at some stage. If you do this (and who can blame you), you will now have eaten the food that your diet suggested in ADDITION to the food you really needed.

So many diets will not work for you because they are forcing you to eat foods that you do not like or enjoy.

There are many reasons why some diets will not work for you, but I don't want to snipe at other diets, I just want you to succeed in your desire to lose weight, which I am sure that you will do if you follow this diet.

WHY IS IT THAT I CAN NEVER STICK TO A DIET?

There are many causes of this problem and most people that are on a diet have trouble sticking with it.

There are many reasons but one of the most common of these is that the diet is forcing you to eat foods that you do not enjoy, or forcing you to exercise etc.

No diet will be fun, you are forcing yourself to eat less and your body will try to prevent this and it will deliberately make you feel uncomfortable. But no diet that is near to torture will succeed for long; it has to stop short of being horrible.

Even a diet like mine that is anything but torture will be hard to follow if there is no instant "payback". But that is exactly what happens with this diet, the hunger sensation is the only discomfort that you will have to put up with and it is hardly torture, but this very same sensation is an instant indication that you are losing weight. This means that you will soon see this sensation as being very positive and you will be happy to know that you are losing weight at that precise moment and so it is no real hardship to feel this for a short while. So on this diet there is no reason why you should not be able to stay with it for as long as you want to.

Any diet that bans your favourite food is also not likely to last that long.

Any diet that turns you into an "obsessive label reader" or a "carrots have zero points" preacher etc. will soon alienate you from your friends, especially at family meal times or "meals out" with friends.

Any diet that relies on you exercising regularly will fail if you are simply not the "exercising type".

Any diet that relies on diet or special foods (cabbage soup - YUK!) will not last, your body needs "proper" food and high quality "fuel" and it will not let you do without these for long.

Any diet that relies on you attending regular meetings or paying for integrated lectures will not last, sometimes you will be simply too busy, you need to be able to have a life!

I will not continue reeling off these reasons why many diets are difficult to follow, I guess that you have already experienced this yourself, or you would not need yet another diet book! But I do honestly believe that you will find this diet VERY different and one that you can follow for as long as you need it.

WHY DO I LOSE WEIGHT AND THEN PUT IT ALL BACK ON AGAIN?

Do you want to have to eat diet foods and avoid "proper" foods for the rest of your life? If so, then any of the "normal" diets may well result in long lasting weight loss.

But if you want to keep the weight OFF and still eat normal foods then you have to find a diet (like this one of course) that achieves the weight loss using foods that you want to be able to eat for the rest of your life.

Let's use a silly example again, let's say we have found a diet that we can follow that claims that we will lose 30 lbs in 4 weeks. All we have to do is to eat nothing but mashed sprouts for the 4 weeks. Now let's just imagine that it worked (it probably would too, I HATE sprouts and so I would starve), at the end of the diet I have now lost my 30 lbs, do I go on eating sprouts - NO! I go back to eating normal foods and so I put the weight back on.

If I had a diet that allowed me to lose weight and still eat normal foods, when I have lost the weight I wanted to lose, I don't have to change anything, I just keep eating normal foods (perhaps just in larger portions if I don't want to keep losing weight). That is why I am sure that you will be able to continue with this diet and not just put the weight back on after you have hit your target weight.

Other reasons for putting weight back on would be if you have selected a diet that does not reduce your stomach capacity. This can often happen on diets that rely on diet foods or low calorie / low points foods, where the volume of the food you are eating increases due to the lack of fuel contained in it.

Your body needs a certain amount of fuel and so if you are eating diet type foods you will have to eat larger volumes of these to get the same fuel as you would from a small portion of "normal" food. So you are NOT reducing your stomach capacity, you are in fact increasing it. The more capacity your stomach has, the more food you will have to eat to feel full. So find a diet that reduces the VOLUME of the food that you eat NOT the amount of fuel in the food you eat (this diet!!!).

If your diet deprives you of certain foods including your favourites such as chocolate, cream, cakes etc., you will crave them more and more and when you have hit your target weight you can often overdo the "treats" and put the weight back on. In this diet you can have these treats occasionally and so at the end of the diet there is no need to dive straight in to your treats.

In all, you need a diet that educates your stomach, reduces it and allows you to enjoy the foods that you are eating. That way, when you hit your target weight, there is no need to change anything, just eat a bit more if you want to stabilise or increase your weight and a bit less to drop it down a bit. You would then be in total control of you weight for ever.

WHY CAN SOMEONE ELSE EAT A LOT AND NOT PUT ON WEIGHT AND I CAN'T?

Firstly, as I have already mentioned several times, we are all different. Our bodies all follow the same basic principles but there are many subtle, but important, differences.

Many of the reasons that we differ in the way that food affects us are caused by habit and lifestyle. If we are used to eating certain foods our body can adapt to those foods over a period of time. If we suddenly eat something completely different, this is new to our body and so it can cause the affect to be different to someone else's if they were used to that food.

For example, I have always eaten lots of chocolate and crisps and so my body is used to processing these foods. It also "knows" that it does not have to store these foods too readily because they are not in short supply. But if someone who hardly ever eats chocolate suddenly eats a bar, their body may decide that it is not a frequent event and therefore it is more likely to store it for use later (i.e. as reserve fat).

I am not saying though, that you should eat lots of chocolate regularly just so that you can eat a bar and not put on much weight!! It is just the way that our body reacts differently to other people and we have to accept that.

What I am saying is that even if you are the type of person who "puts on a pound in weight just when you LOOK at a chocolate bar", you can still have a small portion occasionally. If you feel like some chocolate then have some, but a VERY small portion is all that you need to satisfy your craving (although your body might take a few minutes to realise that you have eaten it).

In summary, we are all different and so don't be surprised if someone else can eat a huge meal and put on no weight and you can't eat a biscuit without "piling on the pounds". What you CAN do, is to educate your stomach to enable it to cope with normal foods without putting on the pounds and by following this diet you should be able to do just that.

IF I DO GET HUNGRY I GET VERY IRRITABLE

I was asked the following question by someone who wanted to try my diet. "If I get hungry, I get irritable and everyone around knows it! Will this diet make me irritable because you encourage me to feel hungry?"

Other people have said EXACTLY the same thing before they tried my diet, (their partners were VERY worried about this "side-effect" of dieting). But all of them have commented that while they were on THIS diet this simply didn't happen.

The difference with this diet when compared to others is that we never "cheat" your body. We respond to the signals that we are getting (after a short period) and give it what it is demanding. This is because when you have felt hungry for a short while, you eat whatever it is that you are craving (in small quantities) rather than tricking your body into thinking that it is being given fuel by eating low calorie "stuff".

When you trick your body like this and give it something other than what it is craving (believe me your body will not send out signals that it wants to eat something that has no "fuel" in it!), it will react and demand even louder for that food that it needs. It is THIS sensation that often triggers what you call irritability, your body is simply sending out such strong warnings that it is preventing you from concentrating on what you are doing and you suddenly develop a very "short fuse".

Eating low calorie foods that trick your body into thinking that it has some "fuel" leave it low on energy and this too can cause you to feel irritable, you must give your body what it is "asking" for, so that it can maintain enough energy to get you through the day.

One tip I would recommend if you do start to become irritable, is to try just sucking a boiled sweet (providing that sugar is not banned for you due to medical reasons, diabetes etc.) to take the edge off the feeling. Remember that eating one boiled sweet will give you a nice burst of energy and it is not going to ruin your diet.

Remember that one of the main elements of this diet is for us to let our body control its own weight; we do this by taking much more notice of the signals that it sends out than we normally do. There should be no need for your body to send out very strong warning signals, if you are following the guidelines and eating "proper" foods that your body is "craving".

If you are still becoming irritable on this diet, it could be due to the fact that you are overdoing the hunger sensation and actually starving yourself. You really must NOT starve yourself, not only is it unnecessary but it will damage your health and you will never stick to the diet. Also remember that I have already pointed out that when you look at how much you weigh now, compared to how much weight you want to lose, this is actually a much smaller percentage than you would think. This means that you don't have to do anything dramatic (such as starve yourself) to get the results you want. So please do not overdo it and you should find that you do not have any problems with irritability.

Stephen Birchall

I NEED MY BREAKFAST AS SOON AS I GET UP EACH DAY.

I was asked about my recommendations for breakfast "This diet recommends that you don't eat breakfast as soon as you get up, but this is when I feel the need to eat more than any other time. I might not be able to follow this rule."

Firstly, I don't like to think of any of the guidelines in this diet as hard and fast "rules". Any diet that tries to force you to do things that you really don't want to do will fail. There is no point in developing a diet that really does help people lose huge amounts of weight if they give up or go back to bad habits because they can't follow all of the "rules". So if you find that there is a guide that you cannot follow, then do not follow it, there are plenty of other guidelines in the book that will help, the more you follow the more weight you will lose, so it is your choice. I am hoping that you will not simply pick and choose the guidelines that you want to follow, but I would be more disappointed (for you) if you didn't follow ANY. But with this guideline, more than most, you can adapt it to suit your own preferences.

I would also suggest that you need to check that you are not causing yourself to feel hungrier than you should feel in the mornings, by doing something else to trigger this. Are you having "midnight snacks" or even waking in the middle of the night and "raiding the fridge / larder"? If you ARE doing this, then this would certainly trigger a hunger as soon as you wake.

Normally when you sleep your stomach processes slow down to a virtual standstill, if they didn't you would experience hunger while you sleep and this would wake you up. If your stomach is still active while you are sleeping then you certainly WILL feel hungry as soon as you wake and you will have to eat something quickly. So what would cause your stomach to be active while you sleep when it should be virtually shut down? Did you eat something just before going to bed? Especially something that was high in fuel or something that had a "slow release" of fuel (such as nuts, cheese etc.)? Eating just before bed is something that is covered by another guideline and it should be avoided if at all possible. This will keep your stomach active and when it has finished processing the food you ate, it will still be active, but with nothing to process! So it will send out the "hunger" signals and wake you up (or at the very least it will make you restless). This will continue through the night and so when you eventually do get up, you will be VERY hungry straight away.

So please do try to avoid eating just before bed and REALLY avoid eating in the middle of the night. Not only are you consuming more food than you need (and so storing it as more fat just when we are trying to get rid of it) but you are keeping your stomach active and so losing sleep to!

If you genuinely feel hungry first thing in the morning, then do eat something or have a drink of tea (or both) if you feel that you have to, but do try not to eat out of habit rather than need. It is so easy to just THINK that you need to eat breakfast just because you have done this all of your life. Remember how we have already talked about the fact that we (as humans) no longer NEED meals anymore? This is especially true of breakfast, we USED TO (as recently as 50 years ago, and that is VERY recent in the history of mankind) HAVE TO fill our stomachs will food to get us through the working day, there were no snacks available. This habit of having to eat meals has been with us for thousands of years, for as long as humans have existed in fact, so it is something that is going to be difficult to change, but we must try if we are to keep healthy.

It is not snacking that causes overweight, it is not even meals that makes us overweight, it is doing BOTH that is the problem. Snacking instead of just having meals is a better option because we do not subject our bodies to too much food to process followed by too little food (just before the next meal). Snacking throughout the day gives us a steady flow of fuel without ever topping up our reserve tank (our fat).

As for the most important meal of the day (possibly?) breakfast, I do have something every morning, but I wait until I get in to work first, before I eat it and only then if I genuinely start to feel hungry enough. That way I am allowing myself to feel the hunger sensation before I eat and this is exactly what we need to do. Eating breakfast just because we have got out of bed and not because we are actually hungry, will result in our body storing it until it needs it and how does it store this? Yes, as FAT.

 But this diet must NOT be torture for you or you will not stay on it. So if you feel like you must have something early in the morning then go ahead and have it. Just try to follow the "Squashable / dilutable" guidelines. One tip to follow is that Muesli and Porridge etc. are not ideal, even though many diets will tell you that they are.

Muesli is too firm and can't be squashed easily (and so breaks our guidelines) this means that it will release fuel throughout the day (which is what most diets recommend) and so stop you from feeling hungry for a long while, but we need to have periods where we feel peckish so that we can lose weight and so I would not recommend Muesli as a good breakfast (as far as dieting is concerned, but do remember that you need to consider your health too, so please eat healthily whatever you eat).

Porridge appears to be squashable and dilutable but the flakes don't actually break down that easily (they just expand in water) they stay intact and are quite firm. Porridge too has a reputation for slow release of energy, which we are avoiding and so I would not recommend having too much.

Having said all this, I still maintain that if you feel hungry for a certain type of food, (even if it is muesli, porridge or toast etc) then go ahead and have it, but just have a small portion. Portion size is far more important than WHAT you are eating.

So have your breakfast and enjoy it, but do try to wait until you are genuinely hungry first.

Stephen Birchall

IF I GO TO BED HUNGRY, I HAVE TROUBLE SLEEPING.

I was asked "Although I agree about not eating last thing in the evening, if I go to bed hungry I have trouble with my sleep pattern, i.e. I go to sleep OK but wake up and I have trouble getting back to sleep. In fact some times I have had to get up in the middle of the night and have something to eat before I can go back to sleep"

It is VITALLY important that you do not give yourself sleep problems, a good restful sleep is so important to your health (mentally and physically). I truly believe that it is far more important to have a good night's sleep than it is to lose a few pounds of weight.

The tip for not eating before bed is not a main guideline; it is just another thing that should help you lose weight. Once again, these are not rules, so if your particular situation means that you cannot follow this then that is fine.

But before you decide that you need to ignore this guideline, think about what may be the real cause of your problem with sleeping. Could it be that there is something else that you need to change? After all, your stomach virtually shuts down when you sleep, so there should be no need for you to eat before you go to bed and certainly not in the middle of the night.

If you are saying that you have to eat before you go to bed or the hunger keeps you awake, then this may be true but a small change in your eating pattern could be all that is needed.

We have discussed the fact, earlier in the book, that your body will take some time to realise that you have eaten something, it has to be swallowed and then the digestion has to break it down, then your stomach has to convert it before your body can tell that it has eaten some fuel. So by eating something just before bedtime will mean that your stomach will be active for some time, especially as it is starting to slow down as you enter the sleep state. This means that instead of getting a deep and relaxing sleep, part of your body (your stomach and whole digestive system) is still working away and is not shut down when it should be. This not only robs you of some of the benefits of sleep, but I wouldn't mind betting that you have plenty of dreams and nightmares as well!

I have a theory about dreams and nightmares and it is relevant to dieting (well almost) and so I don't mind explaining my theory here.

I have discovered over the years that I dream more (much more) if I am uncomfortable in bed. This discomfort could be a new or different bed or bedding or, more often, due to pain. Perhaps I have a small bruise that is tender, an ingrown toenail, mild toothache, a stiff neck etc.

I believe that we dream more when we have a disturbed sleep and that this is caused by the fact that we are constantly moving from a deep sleep to a state where we are almost awake (due to the pain or discomfort etc. as we toss and turn naturally in our sleep) .

I believe that we experience dreams just as we start to wake, which can be very often if we are not in a deep sleep. So if you are having restless nights, the chances are you will be dreaming a lot. The next day you feel as if you haven't really slept.

Now (back to dieting) I also believe that another form of discomfort that can be responsible for causing us to drift from deep sleep to nearly waking, is caused by our stomach being active when it shouldn't be. This would prevent us from staying deep asleep because not everything is shut down, as it should be. This is exacerbated by the body then sending out hunger signals when it has finished processing what we ate just before bed.

This COULD be one of the reasons why people say "don't eat cheese just before you go to bed, it will give you nightmares!" does that sound familiar? I have heard though, that scientists have stated that cheese does NOT give you nightmares and I think that they are probably only partly correct. Cheese in itself may not give you nightmares, but eating something JUST before going to bed could do this. Cheese is very high in fuel and yet it seems to break down slowly and so it would keep your stomach active for a long time while you sleep.

I am sorry if that seemed to be little "off subject", but I do feel that it could be the cause of some sleep problems that people experience, especially those that are associated with food.

If you can manage to have something to eat no later than an hour before you go to bed, than this should be fine. You are aiming to get your timing right so that you are just about to start to feel hungry JUST after you have dropped off to sleep. This means that your stomach will be able to shut down just as you enter a deep sleep and stay shut down until the next day.

Also, be careful about feeling that you have to eat something in the middle of the night to help you go back to sleep (if you wake up). You MAY be thinking that it is eating the food that is helping, but it could be just the fact that you have got out of bed and done something / anything, has helped.

Your stomach should be virtually shut down while you are sleeping or trying to sleep and it would be very rare for it to be sending out signals to get you to eat. In addition to this, the one thing that gives me problems sleeping is when I DO have something to eat just before bed. You body will be trying to process that food and so it will not be going into the "sleep state" until it has finished".

Sleep is SO important for your health and well being, you need to find out what is causing these problems, but I am pretty confident that it will not be lack of food.

Could the problem be caused by the fact that you ARE eating before bed and this is keeping your stomach active, then later on when it has finished processing this food, it is asking for more, because it is still active?

It might be worth trying to eat something an hour before you go to bed at the latest, it COULD be that the food is causing the problem. But don't lose sleep over this!

Weighing myself twice a day will seem odd.

I was also asked "Weighing myself twice a day will seem odd, other diets tell you to weigh yourself weekly or once a day at the very most, why do I need to do this?"

The most important thing that you get from weighing yourself more often and at regular times is that you will be able to work out for yourself the things that increase and decrease your weight. We are all different and it is important for you to discover how YOUR body deals with certain foods. I know, for instance, that when I go to the Chinese for a meal, my weight loss stops for 2 to three days. I also know that this is even worse if I have even the smallest steak or some chicken. You may find different foods affect you differently; this is the only way to make the diet work for you personally. Learn which foods to avoid and also learn how your body gets rid of weight; you can do this by regular and frequent weighing.

After a week or two you will almost be able to guess what the scales will say, and when your guess is wrong, think about what you ate the day before and you will soon figure out what the cause was. Did you have something different, did you have more food than normal or did you drink more, and so on?

Some women have mentioned that their weight alters in line with their monthly cycles and so they believe that they cannot therefore weigh themselves each day. But this should not stop you, the idea is to enable you to know what is happening to your weight and so if you weigh yourself regularly you will soon know what to expect during your cycle and be able to notice weight gains and losses even if your weight varies naturally anyway.

It is important to monitor your weight closely while on any diet, how else will you be able to determine what is working for you, so even though it is not an unbreakable rule, do try to weigh yourself as regularly as you can.

Stephen Birchall

HEALTH

I know that I keep mentioning health throughout the book; it is something that worries me. I hear constantly about health problems associated with dieting. Only yesterday I heard on the news about someone who died because they were using a "water diet" where you are supposed to drink FOUR LITRES of water a day. She drank all four litres within the space of two hours and it killed her. The water in her system caused a problem with her brain.

So I make no apologies about constantly mentioning health throughout the book. If someone can die through drinking too much water then ANY diet has to try to ensure that it cannot lead to any harm to anyone trying it.

I do not want to cause any harm to anyone under any circumstances. I am trying to help people feel better about themselves and become healthier, I do not want to cause ANY problems by any advice I give in this book. But as you will see, if you have read it to here, I avoid any medical suggestions; I do not recommend any food other than "normal" or "proper" foods. I constantly remind you that you must not starve yourself it is totally unnecessary.

If you have any medical problems that require you to eat only certain foods or exclude certain foods from your diet then PLEASE check with your doctor before you go on ANY diet.

I mention sugar a lot in the book and I see this as being a good source of high grade fuel, but if you are diabetic or even suspect that you are, sugar can be very dangerous, once again, if you are not sure, PLEASE check with your doctor before starting ANY diet.

I also tend to mention eating healthily, I avoid specifically recommending which foods you should eat because this varies from person to person, also, if you listen to the "experts" this will vary from day to day and they spend more money in the laboratories analysing and re-analysing their theories.

So eat healthily, read books on the subject of healthy foods and listen to the experts and then make your own mind up as to what is healthy for you and what isn't. Whatever happens, always try to have a balanced diet that includes fruit and vegetables (even if like me you don't like vegetables).

But if you are following this diet correctly you should be using your own body's expert skills to determine what to eat, how much to eat and when. This is the best expert you will ever "listen to".

I have mentioned exercise a lot and I think that there is little doubt that exercise is good for you, but I strongly believe that the AMOUNT of exercise you need will depend on how active you are in your normal life. I cannot see the point of being "super fit" if you sit at an office desk all day and then watch TV all night. More importantly, if this is your lifestyle then you MUST do some exercise to maintain your health.

I certainly do not see any direct link between dieting and exercise, yes if you exercise you will burn up fat, but effectively all that you are doing is ensuring that you are burning up more than you are eating. You can get the same weight loss by just eating less instead and still burn up more than you are eating. In addition to this you are not converting the fat into muscle (which is heavier than fat, you are simply burning it up.

So exercise to stay healthy, do not exercise just because you think it will speed up your weight loss. I am not saying don't exercise just do it for health reasons alone.

If while on ANY diet, watch out for warning signs of any associated problems, especially dizzy spells, headaches and stomach problems. None of these symptoms automatically mean that the diet is the cause, but they COULD indicate that you are overdoing it.

If it is just a feeling that you are a little light-headed, then do eat something with plenty of "fuel" in it, you have probably starved yourself (completely unnecessarily). If this happens more than once, or if you get multiple symptoms together, then do not just assume that it is the diet that is causing them. People on diets are no different to people that are not on diets you can still be struck down by everyday medical problems. Do not just put it down to the diet and miss some early signs that a doctor could pick up and help you with.

All in all, I am saying that you have a responsibility to yourself and those around you to stay healthy, don't let cosmetic changes such as a diet damage your health.

If in doubt check with your doctor, yes they are very busy people and they don't really want people to be taking up their time with fads or imaginary problems, but they would rather see ten cases like that and catch one serious illness early, than miss it altogether.

This is enough of the "negative" aspects of dieting for now, however necessary they are.

EXERCISE

I have already covered this in the previous section "Health" so please read that if you haven't already. But I am torn here as to which message to send out. Exercise is undoubtedly important, but I REALLY don't think that it is an essential part of any diet. So half of me wants to persuade you to exercise but the other half of me wants to persuade you that you don't have to exercise to lose weight.

The basics of exercising to lose weight are fairly uncontroversial; we put weight on when we eat and we lose weight when we exercise and so if we exercise enough to burn up more weight than we put on by eating then YES exercise can help you lose weight. But for me it is easier to change the amount of food that I eat, so that I am eating less than I burn up in my everyday life.

It is not that I am lazy nor is it is that I am against exercise, it is just that for me personally, exercise is BORING and no matter how many times I have tried, I can not keep it up. The effects seem to take so long and the "no pain, no gain" balance means that it is not that enjoyable or endurable.

You may be different and you may well be really "into" exercise, if so, then that is fine and if anything, I am a little jealous. But I believe that any diet that involves exercise is definitely going to fail for ME (and probably many more people too).

So do enough exercise to keep you healthy, try at least to find a nice route to walk regularly (why not get a dog?), or take up golf or some other participation sport that can at least make exercise interesting.

But above all KEEP FIT.

THE BASICS OF THE DIET

This is just a brief summary of the diet for those of you who just want to "cut to the chase". You can read this and get started straight away, then read the rest of the book as and when you want to learn more, especially WHY the diet works.

There are a few theories joined together, based around the fact that our body is an amazing piece of equipment and relying more on the messages from our bodies than diet "experts".

If we can assume that if we over-eat our body stores the extra as fat to use when we miss a meal etc. then we can try to level out our food intake.

Also when our body starts to consume this extra reserve of fuel surely this would feel different, we would surely notice if our body started to consume our fat, there would be SOME sensation? Perhaps this is what we call the sensation we feel when we start feeling hungry? I think this is highly possible.

So this hunger sensation should be seen as something positive, it means that we are able to determine EXACTLY when we are losing weight. So try to allow yourself to feel hungry for a bit longer, don't just eat something "diet" just to take away the hunger.

Golden rules

Golden rule number one is, to eat little and often, this includes meal times. You don't have to give up meals but think of them as a slightly large snack. This is a bit like running a car with only just enough petrol to get you to the next petrol station instead of driving around with a full tank

Golden rule number 2 is, if you are feeling hunger sensations, then you are losing weight. Don't stop the hunger feeling with something low calorie or diet, if it is low calorie or diet then it is not much of a fuel anyway, so why bother. Why not just endure the hunger sensation a bit longer and lose some weight, then eat something that you really want (but not too much)

Golden rule number 3 is, if you are eating a meal, try to eat something that is easily digested and high in water / fluid content. A good guideline is the food should be "squashable" (easily with a fork) and/or dilutable (i.e. contains water / liquid). Foods like this can pass through your digestive system very quickly. Meats and harder foods will stay in your digestive system for a LOT longer (adding to your weight). You can see this happening quite easily, once you start weighing yourself regularly. A meat meal will slow down your weight loss for a day or two at least, a squashable / dilutable meal will be lost almost by the next morning.

Golden rule number 4 is, weigh yourself every night just before bed and then every morning (after having a pee). The morning weights will be your lowest and the evening weights will be the highest. There are two main reasons for doing this, firstly you will get a nice boost each morning because you should be a pound or two lighter than the previous evening and secondly, because you will now be able to see exactly how different foods affect you personally and how long they take to disappear.

Golden rule number 5 is, you MUST be able to enjoy your food and you must NOT starve yourself or miss out on "meals out" or "social meals". To lose weight and keep it off the diet has to be easy to follow and stick to. So if you go out for a meal and really want the steak and all of the trimmings, then HAVE IT!!!!! If you have been following this diet for a while you should have built up some confidence that you are now in control of your weight and so you will know that you will take a small step back but can still lose the extra you will put on.

I personally have started enjoying my food a LOT more since I started this, it seems that the food tastes even nicer and I get more pleasure from eating exactly what I feel like, so you should be able to follow this diet (weight control) for as long as you want to. Which can even be forever, because this diet is all about understanding how to control you weight, not just how to lose it.

Golden rule number 6 is, when you DO eat something eat exactly what you crave (even if this is chocolate, cake etc.) but just watch the quantity (nobody says that you HAVE to finish the whole bar, bag of crisps etc). and your body NEEDS fuel in the form of sugar and fat etc. to operate, you just have to be <u>very</u> careful about the amount you eat.

At meal times just have a large snack instead of a full meal and then snack mid evening a short while after you feel hungry again.

Lesley O, who has tried the diet, has summed it up very nicely as follows

I feel positive that if I eat little and often and allow the hunger sensations to last slightly longer (but not too much) and avoid too much meat and take time to enjoy my food and ensure I eat what I crave then I will lose weight.

Thanks Lesley, I couldn't have put it better myself!

Vegetables / Salads

In many ways, my recommendations for vegetables and salads match my recommendations for exercise. I can absolutely believe that they are good for you, but I personally don't like them. In addition to this, just as with exercise, I do not believe that they should be used as a way to lose weight.

I am a great believer in how "intelligent" your body is and how it let's us know exactly (food wise) what it needs, how much and when. I therefore believe that it is wrong to eat something that your body is not asking for, for any ulterior motive, however good that motive is (dieting for instance).

I personally NEVER feel like vegetables or salads, for some reason, I simply do not like the taste and so I just don't eat them (the nearest I get to vegetables is processed peas and potatoes.) I am fairly sure that the majority of you will disagree and say that you like vegetables and salads, if anything, YOU are "right" and I am "wrong" but that is the way that we are, we are all different.

But as far as a diet is concerned, losing weight should not mean eating something that you do not feel like eating. Diets that tell you to eat plenty of carrots, cabbage, beans, etc., etc. are asking you to ignore the signals from your own body and that cannot be right. If your body is short on salt, for example, then why not eat something salty? Your body was sending those signals for a reason and by ignoring them and eating something else you are "cheating" your body and eating something that is not required. Your body will still need what it was asking for, but you have not eaten it, so you will still be getting the same signals (if not stronger now). This can result in you eating what ever it was that your body was demanding IN ADDITION to whatever your diet told you to eat. If you resist the signals altogether you will find that your body's chemical balance is now harmed and this can lead to mood swings or even leave you open to other problems such as illness etc.

Having said all of this and after stating how much I dislike vegetables and salads, I cannot deny that they are an important food type that we should all be eating. So as far as health reasons are concerned, I fully recommend a BALANCED intake of vegetables and salads. But as far as a diet is concerned, you really should be listening to your body and providing it with what it needs (i.e. eat what you feel like eating, don't trick your body by eating something else just keep the quantity down, especially for high grade fuels such as sugary and fatty foods.)

Diet foods

I include in the category of diet foods, Low calorie, low fat, low sugar, low points and any food that is meant to taste like "real" food but has been modified to remove any natural ingredients.

Firstly we have to look at how these diet foods are meant to help you lose weight. They do this by removing some of the "fuel" from the food, leaving behind some of the taste (perhaps), or they recommend food that has little or no fuel in it to start with.

The idea is based on the simple principal that the less "fuel" that you eat the more weight that you will lose. I can agree with that approach, it is hard to argue against it, but where I disagree and disagree STRONGLY is that I think that it is better to reduce your overall food input to a sensible level by eating less "Proper" food instead of eating the same amount (or more!) of foods with less fuel in them.

One of the main things that many diets try to do is to give you some food options that you can eat to satisfy your hunger without adding too much fuel. But as I have stated many times I firmly believe that allowing yourself to feel hungry is ESSENTIAL to any diet. So for me, diet foods can sometimes be the very reason why you find it difficult to lose weight. You are simply not allowing yourself to feel hungry and so you are preventing your body from burning any reserve fat.

The other problem with diet foods is the volume. If you look at the volume of food needed to provide your body with the right amount of fuel, this volume is MUCH larger if you are consuming lots of diet foods rather than "proper" foods.

If we use an example to illustrate this it may help explain what I mean. If you can agree that your body needs a set amount of fuel to operate and we want this to be low so that we can lose a bit of weight. We can say for this example that you need food with a fuel value of 10 (just an imaginary value). We then have two options for our food, we can eat a small portion of fish with a value of 10 or we can eat a large salad with a value of 8 follow that with a diet yoghurt with a value of 1 and then finish it off with a diet biscuit also with a value of 1.

Which do you think is best if you want to lose weight? You might say that the diet option would be better because the larger volume means that it will satisfy your hunger for longer. Are you sure? Firstly do we WANT to satisfy our hunger for longer? Surely we see the hunger sensation as something that indicates that we are actually losing weight. But more importantly than that, I firmly believe that this is simply not true, both options have the same value and it is the fuel value that satisfies your hunger NOT the volume. Your body sends out the hunger signal when you are running low on fuel and starting to consume your reserves. It does this because it is low on FUEL not low on Volume. So I believe that BOTH will satisfy your hunger for the same duration.

The hidden benefit of the "proper" food is the small size of the portion. IF you can continue to keep the volume of your food low like this, your stomach can start to reduce in size as it gets used to smaller portions and this is VERY positive, in many ways (smaller size means inches lost, it also means a lower capacity so you feel full quicker and also carry less weight in your stomach, MANY benefits!)

But if you feel like the salad INSTEAD of the fish (or whatever option you have available) then fine, this is exactly what I was saying earlier, let your body decide what foods to eat, it is more likely to be able to balance itself correctly.

As for foods that are given a "points" value, I cannot see the POINT of eating a food that has a value of NO POINTS. No points, means no fuel, so why eat it (unless you are eating it to maintain a balanced diet). Eating a large portion of "no point" food can have a doubly negative affect on your weight loss. Not only are you filling your stomach with a high volume of food (just at the time when you want to reduce your stomach), but you are also tricking your body into stopping the hunger sensation while it looks for the fuel in the food you have just eaten.

So I would suggest that you simply try smaller portions of "proper" food instead of large portions of diet foods. There is also the hidden benefit that the cost is likely to be far less if you are avoiding diet foods and just buying smaller quantities of normal foods (and even your shopping bags will lose weight!).

Sugar Chocolate and sweets

I believe that these foods are nowhere near as bad for a diet and many other diets seem to think. They are NOT "taboo" or poison as far as THIS diet is concerned. In fact they are often very useful. Sucking a boiled sweet is a great way of just taking the edge off your hunger when you feel like eating something. The pleasant taste is most welcome after a period of feeling hungry and the sweet turns to liquid quite easily and so does not stay in your stomach for long.

Many "experts" state very clearly that sugar is not by itself fattening and yet most diets tell you to avoid it at all costs. So we need to think long and hard about what it is about sugar, chocolates and sweets that makes it seem so different to other foods.

The main difference about sugar and foods that contain a high volume of sugar is that they are high grade fuels (probably the highest grade fuels you can eat). Sugar gives you LOTS of energy (just ask any mother what it does to their children!). This is the one thing that you have to bear in mind when you are looking at the effects of sugar on a diet (apart from health reasons and the affect on your teeth). If you bear this in mind there is no need to avoid sugar, chocolate and sweets, just be very careful about how MUCH you have.

But why do these harm your diet at all if they are not fattening (according to the experts)? To understand this we need to again think of your body as an engine that needs fuel to drive it. When the fuel is low it switches to the "reserve tank" and starts consuming the extra fat it has stored for this purpose. Sugar being very high in fuel, can provide all the fuel that your body needs for quite a long time, even with the smallest of quantities.

Eat something with a lot of sugar in it and you will have no need to burn off any reserve fat for a long time. This is why it harms your weight loss, it stops you needing to burn off your reserves, it does not add to them as such.

So if you suddenly find that you are craving for something sweet then eat something sweet, because your body is signalling that it needs some energy or that it needs some sugar to balance its chemistry. A classic example of this is when you have eaten a meal you often feel like something sweet; this is why we have developed the habit of having a dessert after a main course. Your body often needs some extra sugar at this point to balance out the savoury food you have just eaten and so you will find yourself often craving something really sweet. Have it, have something sweet, not a diet ice cream have a real ice cream but just one scoop. Better still, have some fresh fruit that is good for your health and your diet and is sweet by nature.

The other problem about sweets and chocolate is the size of the bar or bag. It is VERY tempting to finish the bar or bag and we have built up a habit of doing this over many years. We need to break this habit if we are to lose as much weight as we can.

One tip when eating a chocolate bar is to open the wrapper in a way that it will be easy to cover the remainder of the bar when you have had enough. Just ripping off the top half of the wrapper leaves you with a problem, how can you stop eating it if you cannot cover it up again so that you can finish it later. Sweet manufacturers make the bars that size so that they sell more, it doesn't mean that you have to finish it all in one go.

As for a bag of sweets, a tip here is to again open the bag so that it can be sealed easily later, but then take out just a few sweets and before you start eating them, reseal the bag or fold it over and place it somewhere out of sight. When you have done this, just try that little bit harder to resist opening the bag again until later.

One other danger with sweets and chocolate (in particular) is that because it is very high grade fuel you body will give you rewards to encourage you to eat more. We think of this as being a nice feeling as you are eating it. It simply tastes VERY nice. Your body is rewarding you for eating such a high grade fuel and these rewards are very pleasant. This can mean that at times when you are feeling a bit "low" you might reach for the chocolate or sweets because you want to feel good, not because your body actually NEEDS it. So do take extra care when deciding to eat sugar, chocolate and sweets, male sure that you are ONLY eating it because your body is asking for it, not just because you remember how nice you feel when you eat it.

So if you treat these with caution and eat them ONLY when you REALLY feel you need to, and then only in very small quantities, you should be able to enjoy some every now and then. This may help you stay with the diet; remember I have said many times that it must NOT be torture.

WATER AND DRINKS

Drinks are as important as food in any diet and so you must get this right, but I don't think that you should interfere with your body's own control of the amount that you drink.

Like exercise, I see drinks as being more important from a health point of view than for a weight loss mechanism. You must not drink too little and you must not drink too much. People have died by drinking too little and people have also died by drinking too much.

Your body consists of a huge percentage of water, the actual amount varies depending on the "expert" you consult, but there is no doubt that it forms the major part of your body. This means that you must maintain the right degree of hydration, or you can seriously damage your health.

But I believe, yet again, that your body can indicate very clearly when the balance is wrong. We all experience the sensation of thirst at times and sometimes it is just a mild sensation and other times it is quite strong. Many people don't seem to realise that we also get a sensation that is the opposite of this thirst sensation. We experience this when we have drunk more liquids than we need. This sensation is more difficult to explain and it does not really have a name, but it is just as real.

You may have felt this sensation, especially if you like to drink beer; it manifests itself as a need to eat something dry and or salty. This explains the sale of crisps and peanuts in every bar and pub. It also helps explain the "healthy" (no pun intended) sales of burgers and Kebabs and other "fast" foods near bars and pubs.

Your body senses too much liquid in the system and sends out this signal to encourage you to eat something that will help to soak up or neutralise this excess fluid.

So our body can control its own hydration and we should let it do it and we should not ignore the signals.

Some diets encourage you to drink a LOT of water and many others suggest that you to use it as a means to mask your hunger. You already know what I feel about tricking your body and suppressing the hunger sensation, so I won't expand on this point. But I worry a LOT about anyone drinking large quantities of water when they are simply not thirsty.

Drinking too much has two very basic effects on your weight, firstly every pint of liquid you drink INSTANTLY adds around 1 pound of water (half a litre of liquid adds half a kilo of weight INSTANTLY). This is basic science and so can be taken as fact. Secondly as I mentioned above, if your body senses that you have consumed too much fluid it will send out signals to get you to correct this imbalance. The ONLY way to correct the balance is to eat something dry, salty or something that absorbs liquid.

So basically, drinking too much liquid WILL increase your weight (and also can damage your health remember). The problem is that drinking too LITTLE liquid will also damage your health, so how can we get this right.

My recommendation is quite simple, you should ONLY drink when you are thirsty or when you feel like a drink; do not drink just because you think it will help you to lose weight, or to "flush out your system".

Your body is very sensitive to its fluid balance and your vital organs, such as your kidneys and even your brain rely heavily on this balance being within a narrow range. So you must not become dehydrated or over hydrated just for the sake of adjusting your weight. There is no simple formula and even the recommended levels from "experts" vary. Add to this the added complexity due to the amount of fluid that most foods contain anyway, the salts you take in and the effect of perspiration and you can see that it is a very difficult thing to manage. But if you trust your body and the signals it gives, then you will not go far wrong.

I would also recommend using scales that can indicate your water content. I have deliberately not included any charts to indicate what to aim for because I will leave this to the medical experts.

So to summarise, drink when you feel like drinking, do not drink more than you need and look after your health THEN your weight.

BREAD

At first this would appear to be OK because it appears to be squashable and dilutable, but unfortunately its effect can be very negative when it comes to weight loss.

When I was developing this diet I believed it to be OK because it APPEARS to be within the guidelines. But the results of the regular weighing seemed to indicate otherwise.

The first time I noticed this was when I had soup, which is a great food on this diet, full of fuel and almost liquid. The next day I didn't seem to lose as much weight as I had expected, it wasn't much different, but enough to make me wonder. I had three slices of bread with my soup and felt that this would not make much difference, the weight of three slices is not much and it looks like it could be easy for the stomach to break down. A few days later and I experienced the same thing; the only explanation was that the bread was the cause. I continued to experiment and found the same kind of problem when I ate sandwiches. It became clear that the bread was somehow causing the weight loss to reduce slightly.

To fully match the squashable / dilutable guidelines the food should come apart slightly when squashed, bread tends to just spring back into shape. As for the dilutable test, yes bread can be diluted but all it does is to swell up and not break down at all. So even though it appears to match the guidelines it actually doesn't quite.

I think that the main problem is more due to the effect that the bread has on other foods in the stomach. It soaks them up and holds them like a sponge, turning pure liquid foods into semi solid.

This results in the food staying in the stomach a little longer and so enabling the stomach to extract more "fuel" from it and preventing it from being expelled via urine.

This does not mean that bread should be avoided altogether but it does mean that you should perhaps reduce the amount of bread that you eat slightly. Still have a slice of toast as your first snack if you want to, but try not to have two and bread rolls and sandwiches are not great.

Pies, Pastries and Cakes

I think that you may be able to guess the recommendations for this type of food? They are likely to hold up your weight loss if eaten in any quantity, but do remember that you can eat whatever you feel like, just keep the portion size down.

The worst option of these that you could select would be a meat pie of any description, the combination of the meat, the gravy and the pie itself mean that it would hold up your weight loss for a day or two (depending on how much you eat of course). But not all pies are that bad, a cheese and onion pie or most pies that do not contain meat or chicken should be ok in sensible portions.

Pastries and cakes can obviously be fattening, but if you are getting the signals from your body that you need to eat something sweet and dry, then a small portion of cake or a small pastry is fine. Also remember that you have to feel that you can stick to this diet and the odd treat is a great way of achieving this.

If anything, a small cake covered in chocolate or icing is probably better than a larger portion of a basic sponge cake (remember the section on the volume of food for the same amount of fuel).

So enjoy your treats, I am pretty sure that you will find that ALL food tastes nicer on this diet because you are always eating what your body is asking for and you will savour every mouthful.

Soups

This is my favourite snack type food of all, it is tasty, comes in so many varieties and often in just the right size.

I tend to use it in place of a full meal, with one slice of bread. I can eat it and yet still feel a little peckish when I have finished, PERFECT!

I like the "chunky" soups, they are close to a meal and yet they squash so easily. Even the soups that have meat in them normally have it as small pieces and there is not a lot of meat anyway.

So if you enjoy soups, you can have them as and when you feel like, as long as you have been following all of the other guidelines.

Don't go for the low calorie soups, they may not provide enough fuel for your needs and you may need to eat again after a short while anyway, destroying the "benefits" of the lower calories anyway.

Stephen Birchall

Nuts

There are many different types of nuts but they mainly have the same effect on your weight. I would not avoid nuts, they are a good source of fuel, in fact they are so rich in fuel that you have to be careful and don't have too many.

You may find that you often feel like having some salted peanuts after having a few drinks, this is fine, it is just your body's way of balancing out the fluids you have been drinking.

Do observe the "eat slowly" guideline, though, especially when eating salted nuts, it is surprising how little salt you may need and it will take a while before your body registers that you have eaten any.

Nuts are not that dilutable but they do break down relatively easily when crushed and so they are not a bad snack. The fact that they are a high grade fuel means that you don't have to eat a large volume to provide your body with plenty of energy, this works well because we are trying to reduce the volume of food that we eat.

In many ways the recommendations for sugar match those for nuts, they have a very similar effect on your weight.

So if you enjoy the occasional packet of nuts, this is not a problem, just try to break the habit of eating a whole packet.

Potatoes

These certainly fit in with the guidelines, they are very easily squashed and easily diluted, and in fact mashed potato is exactly that, squashed and diluted potatoes!

At mealtimes, even if you are aiming to just have a snack, such as a piece of fish and some vegetables, you can certainly add some potatoes as long as this doesn't result in too large a snack.

Keep the volume of chips down to a minimum and try not to have roast potatoes (dry roast potatoes are fine though, have you tried these?).

Boiled, steamed, mashed and jacket potatoes are ideal and can be a regular food in small portions. They have a reasonable amount of fuel in them and your stomach can break them down very easily. Their high water content means that most of the weight can be lost via urine very quickly after you have eaten them.

I am a big potato fan, I REALLY like the taste, probably a bit too much, which means that I often eat slightly more than I should, but this is not a problem for me, I know that I can still lose weight on this diet and so the effect of the potatoes is not a problem.

I have switched away from chips (I used to eat FAR too many chips) and now my favourite potatoes are steamed new potatoes. The steaming seems to retain more of the flavour. In fact, in all honesty I actually prefer my steamed new potatoes to chips and I NEVER thought that I would say that.

Baked potatoes are good, especially if you replace one of your meals with a baked potato and a light filling (some butter is fine and so is cheese, beans etc.) but do not have meat or chicken fillings if you can manage to avoid them.

I would suggest that you try rice for a couple of meals a week and potatoes for a couple of other meals and do without either on the remaining meals. Although hopefully the meals you are having are just large snacks?

Fats and Butter etc.

Almost all diets and many medical experts point out the "dangers" of fats and so I am not going to repeat this here, but it is fair to say that you MUST be careful about how much fat you eat.

Once again I will not give you specific medical advice, I will leave that up to the experts, PLEASE do read the many articles that have been written on the subject.

As far as losing weight is concerned, fats are one of the high grade fuels but with a sting in the tail!

Imagine the process your body has to go through to convert your food into fat that is stored as reserve fuel. This is quite a task and the one thing that we need to avoid is anything that makes this task easier! It is VERY easy for your body to convert fat into fat. So whatever you do, do not overeat anything that contains fat.

You don't have to avoid it altogether, your body NEEDS fat as a fuel, just be sensible.

If you do decide to eat any meat (and hold up your weight loss for a few days) then please try to eat lean meat. Cut off any visible fat, skin, gristle, rind etc. and eat only the lean part of the meat. Don't make it easy for your body to put back the fat that you have worked so hard to burn off.

Butter on bread is fine (a thin coating) and there is no need to only eat low fat foods from a WEIGHT LOSS point of view (but listen to the medical advice).

We are going to be letting our body control its own weight and so if we eat a small amount of fat we should not feel hungry for a bit longer than usual and this should self-regulate our eating habits.

Creams and custards etc. fall into the same category and the same advice applies.

Milk is different, this is a liquid and even in full fat milk there is not going to be much left for the body to store, but remember that the fat in milk can be easily stored so if you can use low fat milk it is better, but milk, in general is fine. I would certainly not suggest that you leave milk out of your coffee, teas etc. a splash of milk is tiny in relation to your weight.

With all of the fats and similar foods just be very careful that you do not overdo it by having many different parts of your meal that all contain fat, the cumulative effect could be a problem. For example, a piece of chicken, with the skin on, coated in cheese and covered in gravy, followed by a dessert with custard and a milky coffee, will not just delay your weight loss, it will increase your weight very quickly. But each item by itself is fine.

Meat and Chicken

No food on this diet is banned but if it was, it would be meat and chicken. This is the one thing that will delay your weight loss and even possibly add weight.

Having said this, if you are NOT a vegetarian I would think it would be very difficult for you to completely give up meat and chicken, so you can have it if there is no other choice or if you are enjoying a meal out and don't want to be a "party pooper". But if you seriously want to lose weight it is the one thing that will help most.

Meat and chicken are NOT squashable and NOT dilutable and so your stomach will take a LONG while to process it. This results in two problems, firstly while the meat or chicken is still in your stomach, it is included in your body weight, secondly because it is in your stomach for a long time your body can continue to take fuel from it over a long period. This also enables your body to store the excess as fat.

So if you were to cut out meat and chicken altogether, you will be able to obtain the maximum benefit of this diet.

I am a big meat lover, I REALLY enjoy a good steak, but I would prefer to do without this pleasure to some extent, to get to my target weight. In fact, I have a very real and very serious dilemma. I love meat and I love animals. I have tried to become a vegetarian in the past, even though I don't like vegetables!!!! I simply didn't want to be responsible for any animal suffering. I am not preaching here, just explaining my feelings.

This attempt at becoming a vegetarian did not last long, my diet was too restricted, I did not like vegetables or salads and so I was limited to cheese, soups, dairy products, desserts etc. This was a very unbalanced diet and so I was soon experiencing light headedness, stomach pains and a general feeling of malaise. Reluctantly I started to eat meat again and felt very guilty (even though I still enjoyed the taste to be perfectly honest.)

One by-product of this diet is that I have slowly managed to cut down my meat intake to virtually nil (just special occasions only). I have certainly not become a vegetarian, I eat a lot of fish and seafood now and on certain occasions I will have a small piece of meat or chicken but I am very pleased to have at least dramatically reduced my meat intake.

So avoid meat and chicken if you want to gain the full benefits of the diet, but special occasions or after you have hit your target weight, you can start eating small portions of meat or chicken if you really want to.

FISH

On this diet I now eat far more fish than I ever used to and I really believe that this has had benefits apart from losing weight.

When I used to go out for a meal, which I do quite often, I only ever seemed to opt for the steak or meat. I even rarely went for the chicken option. I simply enjoyed my meat too much to choose anything else, after all, if I am having a treat I want my favourite food, I wouldn't experiment with other foods just in case I didn't enjoy it and therefore spoil my treat.

I was quite happy doing this and it would be very rare for me to choose fish as a special treat, not because I didn't like fish, it was just that I didn't see it as "special".

Now I am on this diet meals out are even more of a treat, I have broken my "meat habit" and I now try the other options that I have up until now, avoided. This means that I now go for the fish option more often than not. It could be Fisherman's pie, the sea food platter, a nice sea bass etc. etc. I even switched to eating a lot of Sushi, especially as a lunchtime snack.

So my diet is now far more varied than it has ever been and a lot more fun.

Fish does match the squashable guideline, it can be squashed very easily and breaks down when you eat it. But it does not match the dilutable guideline, it is cannot be diluted, which I guess is just as well if you are a fish!!!

Stephen Birchall

Fish is a great food, there is a fair amount of fuel in it, but not too excessive and your stomach can process it very quickly. So fish is great, try to include it is many snacks, this is especially easy due to the huge variety you have available.

One fish option that could be a small problem is the firmer fish meals such as tuna or swordfish steaks. These have a texture very similar to meat and so will stay in your stomach for a long while. They are not as bad as meat but they are not as good as the other fish based meals, they are not easily squashed. Other forms of tuna etc. are fine, it is a tasty and nourishing food and works well with baked potatoes and salads.

So if you enjoy fish, use it often in your diet, they say that it is good for your health too. If you do not enjoy fish, perhaps you should give it a try, there are many different types of fish and you may find one that suits you.

DESSERTS

Just the mention of the word "desserts" makes my mouth water, I am a confirmed "sweet" person, I LOVE deserts.

But they are so high in fuel and you are eating them after already having a main course, they will slow down your weight loss.

If my will-power is strong and I am having a meal out or with friends, I can leave out the dessert and so instantly cut down on the volume of fuel that I eat. But if I REALLY feel like a dessert I order a small ice cream. This breaks down into liquid very quickly and so is easily expelled just as quickly.

Other desserts such as pies, pastries, cakes and more solid options are to be avoided, not only are they high in fuel but they will take a long time to digest too.

The problem with desserts is that they are necessary, your body does "ask for them" after a meal. I often have a meal (large snack) and soon after I find myself craving something sweet. Your body is simply trying to balance itself again and the sweetness compensates for the savoury meal you have just eaten, After all, that is why desserts are eaten after the meal anyway.

One option I go for is to leave out the dessert and get my sweetness from the after-dinner mints and coffee (sweetened).

So if you are eating out and you really want to treat yourself to a full main course, rather than go for a "more sensible" option,, have your choice and miss out on the dessert instead.

Beer, wine and spirits

Strangely enough, most, if not all, experts will tell you that these drinks, by themselves, are not fattening. This is not as surprising as it seems, after all, they are simply liquids and your body can get rid of them very quickly. They do not contain any fat or sugar (apart from in any mixer you add to them) and so why are they such a problem.

Why do we see so many "beer bellies" if the beer is not fattening?

Two things are causing this.

Firstly the fact that your body will try to balance out all of that liquid by making you crave dry and salty foods, foods that you would not have normally eaten.

Secondly, the sheer volume of all of that liquid will have stretched your stomach and probably by a lot if you are a heavy drinker. This increase in stomach size will obviously increase your "belly" size and what is worse; it will have increased your stomach capacity, so it will now take more food to make you feel full.

Wine and spirits have the same effect but the volumes involved tend to be smaller, although drinking a bottle or two of wine will certainly stretch your stomach.

Spirits are normally mixed with fruit juices and cola etc., this increases the volume and can also increase the sugar content.

But one of the biggest effects on your weight loss will be due to the fact that while you are drinking, your stomach will not be consuming your reserve fat, it will be too busy dealing with the drinks. It will not be sending out the hunger signals because it has something to process.

Remember also that one litre of fluid weighs one KILO of weight, so having a lot to drink will increase your weight (at least temporarily) and it will do this INSTANTLY.

So it is a good idea to reduce the volume of alcohol to as low as you feel you can manage. This will not only help you with your weight loss but it will certainly help you with your health.

CHEESE

As long as you consider the fact that cheese is another high grade fuel, there is no need to avoid it altogether. I eat a cheese quite often, it has a lot of flavour and it is easily squashed.

I really enjoy cheese and I have found that apart from just reducing the amount slightly, I can carry on enjoying it and the many different types available.

One of my favourite mealtime "snacks" is a three egg, cheese omelette. I find that I can eat this and still feel peckish afterwards, which is perfect.

Like many other foods, you will sometimes have a craving to eat some cheese, but this does not seem to happen very often and so you can normally have it as and when you feel like it. If you want to accompany it with "crackers" or other biscuits designed for cheese, that should be ok, just stop before you get anywhere near feeling full and you should not have had too much of an effect on your weight loss.

I see cheese as a treat and it is important to still have treats even though you are on this diet.

The high grade fuel in cheese means that it can be ideal after feeling hungry for a while; it should ease that feeling until you are ready to lose a bit more weight.

PASTA

Pasta contains a LOT of water, you can see this when you look at dried pasta and realise just how much it swells when cooked.

This makes it a perfect choice when eating out or for a mealtime snack at home. Eat it with little or no meat (try seafood or just vegetarian options) and you will find that your weight loss is hardly affected.

I have become a regular at our local Italian restaurant since I have started this diet; I have yet to have a "nasty surprise" from the scales after eating normal sized portions of pasta, sometimes in larger portions that I had planned even.

I can even have a starter of Minestrone soup as well as a pasta main meal and still follow the guidelines of my diet.

So if you like pasta, enjoy it whenever you want to and still lose weight.

Why not try using Soya or Quorn based meat substitutes, they are perfect when added to an Italian sauce to make a meat free Bolognese or Lasagne. You still get the flavour and texture but without the penalties.

A TYPICAL DAY

The following is one example of what I would call a typical day on this diet. Remember that this is a very flexible diet and so this is just a guide it should not be seen as a set of instructions. But if you just want to start off by trying the diet first before you read all of the details in the book, then this will at least give you a starting point.

Your day may be very different to someone else's day (for example a hard working mum with young children to look after, is going to have a very different day to someone who is stuck in an office all day, or a bus driver, gardener, doctor etc.). But whatever your day is like you should be able to use the following as a guide.

— First thing in the morning, before you get dressed, weigh yourself, after a pee, remember one litre of fluid weighs one kilo (just over 2 lbs)). This gives you a stable weight measurement to enable you to monitor how you are doing (If you are female you may find that your weight naturally alters in cycles throughout the month, but this is fine, after a while you will be able to allow for this).
If this is not the first day of your diet and you have not lost anything since your weigh-in last night, remember what you ate yesterday and see if there is a reason for this and learn from that (did you eat any meat or anything else that is not squashable / dilutable?, or drink a lot of fluids?).
If it is your first weigh-in on this diet then remember this weight, you should use this as your starting point. This should be your lowest weight of the day and so we can genuinely tell if you are losing weight when you weigh yourself the next morning.

- This is VERY important; don't just assume that you have to eat breakfast just because you have just got out of bed. You may not actually be THAT hungry, it could be that you are eating breakfast at this time just out of habit.

  Whenever you eat something it should be because you are hungry and do not want to feel the hunger sensation any longer, you must not just eat because of the time of day etc.

  There is no problem with having a cup of tea, coffee, juice, milk etc. that is fine, after all it is merely flavoured liquid and so is not going to cause you to put on weight for long (at least only until the next visit to the toilet for a pee!) but only have something to eat if you really feel very hungry and have something that you are craving, as along as it is not Bacon, sausage etc, with all of the trimmings, unless you don't mind delaying your weight loss for a day or two?.

  Toast (with butter and jam / marmalade etc. is fine but try just having one slice of toast.

  The squashable / dilutable guide applies equally here, as it does to anything you eat, so egg is fine, bacon is not, tomatoes are fine, fried bread is not (have you ever tried to dilute grease?).

  But do remember that you do not have to feel full after your breakfast, you can always have a snack later in the morning when you have to. A large breakfast will be stored by your body for release later on and we are trying to REVERSE the fat we have stored not ADD to it.

- Throughout the day you will obviously start to feel hungry, if you really want to lose weight then this is the time when the diet can work best for you.

  See this "hunger sensation" as the feeling you will get when your body is consuming the fat it has stored.

  This means that the LAST thing that you should do when you start to fell hungry is to immediately eat something (even if this is zero calories, zero points, or even water) we WANT to experience this sensation or we are simply not losing any weight. So see this as a clear indication that your diet is working and at that precise moment in time your ARE losing weight.

When you have felt hungry for a short while and you start to feel uncomfortable (under no circumstances leave this too long, you do not have to starve yourself), have a snack of whatever you want. This CAN be a diet or low calorie snack, but why bother eating something if it is not giving your body the fuel you need, you will just feel hungrier later anyway.

I would prefer you to use your body's abilities to indicate what it needs and therefore eat something that you are craving. If this is something savoury, then eat something savoury, if this is something sweet, then eat something sweet, (dry, liquid, hot, cold etc. etc.) but most importantly eat a small portion of it rather than your "normal" amount. Remember the aim is just to eat enough to maintain your health and energy, we must not eat to feel full or we will simply be storing MORE fat as reserves. Remember that if you can eat whatever it was you felt like but still feel a bit "peckish" afterwards then this is perfect. You have eaten what your body wanted and are still losing weight.

But (sorry for repeating myself, but it is very important) you must NOT starve yourself, remember that to lose the weight you have set as your target you do NOT have to DRAMATICALLY change your eating habits, you just need to reduce the volumes that you eat. Reducing your food intake too much can lead to serious health issues and it is completely unnecessary, you can still lose the weight you want to even if you just reduce your food intake a little at first.

- Keep this up during the day, allowing yourself to feel "peckish" for longer than you normally would.
  In these modern times we have access to good quality, healthy snacks throughout the day.
  If you really do not have access to snacks during the day due to your lifestyle / job, then do try to have a packet of something that you can eat to prevent you from feeling too hungry, instead of filling yourself up at mealtimes (and therefore storing more fat).
  Remember that it is vital to have a balanced diet and so try to vary the snacks you have (let you cravings tell you what your body needs and eat a small amount of what you crave)

- At lunch time / evening meal time, have a meal if you want to, but try to make it a large snack rather than filling up.
  You do not have to sit separately from your fiends and family or avoid food at mealtimes; just make sure that you just have a snack sized portion.
  Meals can be an important social event and so you must not be seen as a slave to your diet, you also have to enjoy your diet and you won't if you find yourself feeling remote from everyone around you.
  If you decide to have a meal rather than a snack, then that is fine, there are no hard and fast rules to this diet, juts remember that the best foods for your diet should be easy for your stomach to process (so that they can come out again very quickly). So try to eat foods that are squashable / dilutable so that they are not stored in your body for any longer than they need to be.
  Be careful of the volume of food you eat at mealtimes, but do not go for low calorie or diet foods, this will just trick your stomach into thinking that it has been given some fuel and you will just feel hungrier later and so be tempted to eat more anyway.
  I personally do not like salads (or even vegetables) but if

you really do enjoy these then have them, they form part of a balanced diet, but do not eat them out of habit. If your body does not crave them then it may well not need them at every meal.

Remember that this diet is all about losing weight and you don't need salads or vegetable to lose weight, but YOU DO need them for health reasons so please do follow all of the medical advice and eat healthily, but do not see these foods as a key to losing weight, they are NOT. Having a snack at mealtime that does not fill you is perfect, once again you will have given your body the fuel that it needs by eating the food that it craves and yet you may still feel a bit peckish afterwards, This is what we are aiming for, remember that the "hunger sensation" is a clear (and instant) indication that you are losing weight, so if you have eaten healthily and still feel peckish this is a "Win Win" situation.

You can always have a snack later if you need to, you don't have to fill your stomach just because it is meal time. Get this right and you are well on your way to your target weight.

— Snack throughout the rest of the day / evening whenever you feel that you want to ease the "hunger sensation" but do try to experience it for a short while at least.

Do try to avoid a late snack (just before bed), the main reason for this is that if you are asleep you won't notice your hunger sensations. So if you go to bed a bit peckish then this is great (don't leave yourself so hungry that it could keep you awake).

But whatever you do, don't go to bed feeling full, your body will have all night to process every piece of that food and convert it to fat reserves.

Your body does not consume much of your fat reserves overnight either. The reason I say this is because when you wake up you never seem to be hungrier than when you went to sleep. Could this be because your body shuts down this consumption of fat because you are not burning much energy while you are asleep? I think that this is entirely possible and this is yet another reason why I say that you should not have breakfast as soon as you wake up. You may not be feeling hungry and so if you eat something just out of habit, your body may well store more of this as fat reserves.

– Weigh yourself just before bedtime to see how your weight has been affected by the food that you have eaten all day, but don't be too disappointed if you have not lost anything since the morning weigh-in, after all you have eaten and had drinks and this is still in your stomach (or at least most of it is) and it all has weight, so you are likely to be a fair bit heavier than you were this morning.
But the nice thing is that you should lose a pound or two by morning whatever happens because you will lose fluids (via sweat) and urine before your morning weigh-in.
This is one of the reasons I like to weight myself morning and night, virtually every morning I can see the scales going in the right direction. Not only that but if your weight in the morning is the same or worse than it was the previous morning then you should be able to tell why that is. Was it because you decided to eat something that was not that squashable / dilutable, or did you have a full meal (not a problem but it would explain why), or did you have a lot to drink? Whatever happens, use these regular weigh-ins to determine exactly what works for YOU and hopefully they will give you that boost of seeing your weight reducing and help you keep it up.

THE GOLDEN RULES

These are the main rules to follow if you want this diet to work for you, once again, these are not rules that MUST be followed this diet does not work that way (no diet would). It is just that to get the most benefit from the diet you should understand these golden rules and try to follow them as closely as possible.

Golden rule number 1 is, to eat little and often, this includes meal times. You don't have to give up meals but think of them as a slightly large snack. This is a bit like running a car with only just enough petrol to get you to the next petrol station instead of driving around with a full tank This is nothing new, lots of diets work on the principal of "little and often" but few explain the logic behind this. Hopefully you have read the section where I explain about this and where I talk about why we do not necessarily need meals anymore. One side-benefit of eating little and often is that your stomach will soon adjust to the smaller volumes of food and so you will gradually need less food to feel full anyway.

Golden rule number 2 is, if you are feeling what we call "hunger" sensations then you are losing weight. This sensation that we call "hunger" is actually felt because your body is consuming the fat it has built up in reserves instead of using the contents of your stomach. We only THINK that it is a signal to eat food (which it would be if we were at our target weight). So you should see this as a very positive sensation if you are on a diet. You can use it as an <u>instant</u> indication of when you are losing weight. Because of this you should not rush to stop the hunger feeling by eating or drinking low calorie or diet (if it is low calorie or diet then it is not much of a fuel anyway, so why bother?). Why not just endure the hunger sensation a bit longer and lose some weight, (and KNOW that you are losing weight) you can then eat something that you really want (but not too much) later when you feel that you don't want to feel the sensation any longer.

Golden rule number 3 is, if you are eating a meal, try to eat something that is easily digested and high in water / fluid content. A good guideline is the food should be "squashable" (easily with a fork) and/or dilutable (i.e. contains water / liquid), ideally BOTH. Foods like this can pass through your digestive system very quickly. Meats and harder foods will stay in your digestive system for a LOT longer (adding to your weight). In addition to this the longer the food stays in your digestive system the more energy / fat your stomach can extract and save. You can see this happening quite easily, once you start weighing yourself regularly. A meat meal will slow down your weight loss for a day or two at least but a squashable / dilutable meal will be lost almost by the next morning (or the next pee!). One extreme example of this is as follows; A half litre of water weighs the same as a half kilo of steak, so the immediate weight gain from both is half a kilo !!! The BIG difference is that the water can be passed out again VERY quickly (as pee) but the meat will take a long while to process, so a few hours later the weight from the water will be gone, but the weight from the steak will still be there. So basically if the food is squashable and or dilutable, your body can process it quicker. So if you have a choice of meal, bear this in mind and you can still have a complete wholesome meal without damaging your weight loss too much. There is a list of foods elsewhere in the book and this gives plenty of examples.

Golden rule number 4 is, weigh yourself every night just before bed and then every morning (after having a pee). The morning weights will be your lowest and the evening weights will be the highest. There are two main reasons for doing this, firstly you will get a nice boost each morning because you should be a pound or two lighter than the previous evening and secondly, because you will now be able to see exactly how different foods affect you personally and how long they take to disappear.

Golden rule number 5 is, you MUST be able to enjoy your food and you must NOT starve yourself or miss out on "meals out" or "social / family meals". To lose weight and keep it off, the diet has to be easy to follow and stick to. So if you go out for a meal and really want the steak and all of the trimmings, then please have it, it will not be a disaster for your diet it will just delay the weight loss for a few days. If you have been following this diet for a while, you should have built up some confidence that you are now in control of your weight and so you will know that you will take a small step back but can still lose the extra you will put on. Not only should you enjoy your meals out, but I firmly believe that you will start to enjoy all of your food more once you have started this diet. I personally have started enjoying my food a LOT more since I started this, it seems that the food tastes even nicer and I get more pleasure from eating exactly what I feel like. This is mainly because I am allowing myself to feel hungry for a bit longer before I eat, but also because I eat smaller quantities of my favourite foods and so really enjoy the flavour more because I am not overdoing it (you CAN have too much of a good thing). So this means that you should be able to follow this diet (weight control) for as long as you want to, which can even be permanent, because it is all about understanding how to control you weight, not just how to lose it.

Golden rule number 6 is, when you DO eat something, eat exactly what you crave / fancy (even if this is chocolate, cake etc.), but just be careful about the quantity (nobody says that you HAVE to finish the whole bar, bag of crisps etc). Your body NEEDS fuel in the form of sugar and fat etc. to operate, you just have to be <u>very</u> careful about the amount you eat. Trust your body and eat what your body seems to be telling you to eat.

So if you do nothing else and just understand the above golden rules, at least you will know how to control your weight (whether you do or not is entirely up to you)

THANK YOU

Please accept my sincere thanks for buying this book and trying my diet.

I am very confident that, if you have followed most of the guidelines and tips, you will have been able to improve your weight, health and wellbeing.

I always welcome feedback of all kinds and you can visit my web site www.TheBirchallDiet.com if you want to pass on any messages. I would especially like to hear any success stories, not merely to try and boost sales, I GENUINELY want to hear that I have been able to help people feel better about themselves.

There will be a forum for people to discuss dieting and a few helpful links, so please do visit.

Keep the book handy so that you can always use it if the scales start to show any movement in the wrong direction.

I wish you all the best in whatever you do.

THANK YOU.

Steve Birchall

Lightning Source UK Ltd.
Milton Keynes UK
06 January 2010

148227UK00002B/18/P